'A marvellous memoir on the human side of GP practice ... His resolutely non-specialist memoir may, I think, turn out to be one of the classics which every medical student *must* read. ... I don't think anyone since AJ Cronin has expressed so strongly what it is to be embedded in the community as a GP.'

Libby Purves,
BBC Radio 4 *Midweek*

'I simply could not put down this extraordinary mixture of stories from the GP's surgery in suburban London. ... Two clear messages emerge from this book, which should be required reading for every medical student. ... First, medicine must relearn its heart and soul ... Second, there is no certainty in medicine, and no clear answer as to what it is that cures, or fails to cure people. ... Clearly told, and an extraordinary read, this is a passionate cry for humane medicine.'

Dame Julia Neuberger,
The Independent

D1353908

Also by the author

Doctors and Patients: an anthology
(2002)

Culture, Health and Illness, 4th edition
(2001)

The Body of Frankenstein's Monster:
Essays in Myth and Medicine
(1992)

Body Myths
(1991)

The Golden Toenails of Ambrosio P
(1990)

Prose Poems

Irregular Numbers of Beasts and Birds
(2006)

The Girl on the Aeroplane
(2002)

The Exploding Newspaper & Other Fables
(1981)

Suburban
Shaman
tales from medicine's frontline

To my daughter Zoe

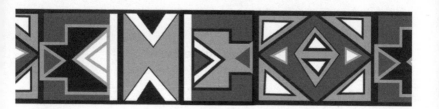

Suburban
Shaman
tales from medicine's frontline

Cecil Helman

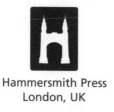

Hammersmith Press
London, UK

First published 2004 in southern Africa by Double Storey books,
a division of Juta & Co Ltd, Cape Town, South Africa.

First published in Great Britain 2006 by Hammersmith Press Limited,
496 Fulham Palace Road, London SW6 6JD, UK
www.hammersmithpress.co.uk

Author's note
Where I have included case histories, descriptions of patients, or dialogue, usually
recreated from memory after many years or even decades, I have taken considerable
care in each case to protect the identity of the people involved. I have changed a variety
of medical, personal, historical and other identifying details, including sometimes the
time, place and circumstances of the encounter – in some cases blending similar stories
together. Despite this occasional but very necessary 'fictionalisation' to protect identity,
every single one of the case histories is based originally on real people and on real
events. I am very grateful to the people concerned, and I hope that I have described
them with the respect and compassion that they deserve. I am also confident that
anyone who thinks they recognise themselves in a case history will be mistaken, for I
have deliberately selected stories that are in some ways archetypal, with each one
representing many hundreds of very similar cases: the types of case that would be
familiar to any family doctor, in almost every practice in the land.

British Library Cataloguing in Publication Data:
A CIP record of this book is available from the British Library.

ISBN 1-905140-08-8

Designed by Amina Dudhia
Typeset by Julie Bennett
Production by Helen Whitehorn, Pathmedia
Printed and bound by TJ International Ltd of Padstow, Cornwall, UK

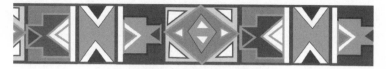

CONTENTS

ACKNOWLEDGEMENTS

I would like to acknowledge the following sources that I have quoted in this book. Full details of the original publications are given in the Bibliography.

Arthur Conan Doyle's quotation is from *Tales of Adventure and Medical Life* (John Murray, 1963). Rachel Naomi Remen's quotation is from *My Grandfather's Blessings: Stories that heal* (Riverhead Books 2000). Saul Bellow's quotation is from *Mosby's Memoirs and Othe Stories* (Weidenfeld & Nicholson, 1969). Susan Sontag's quotation is from *Illness as Metaphor* (Penguin, 1991). Anaïs Nin's quotation is from *Winter of Artifice* (Peter Owen, 1974). Oliver Sacks's quotation is from *A Leg to Stand On* (Picador, 1984). I.M. Lewis's quotation is from *Ecstatic Religion* (Penguin, 1971). Franz Kafka's quotation is from the story *Ein Landarzt*, first published in German in Leipsig in 1919. Roy Porter' quotation is from *The Cambridge Illustrated History of Medicine* (Cambridge University Press, 1966). Mircea Eliade's quotation is from Masks: mythical and religious origins, in *Symbols, the Sacred and the Arts*, edited by Diane Apostolas-Cappdona (Crossroads, 1986). The quotation from JAMA is from L.D. Grouse's Editorial, Has the machine become the physician? (*Journal of the American Medical Association* **259**, 1891).

Every effort has been made to trace copyright holders. The publishers will be happy to correct mistakes or omissions in future editions.

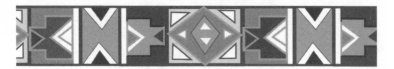

INTRODUCTION

I come from a family of 13 doctors and not a few hypochondriacs. Among my relatives I can also count a medical librarian, a medical researcher, a medical secretary, a medical social worker, and a technician in a medical laboratory. In fact, the family connection with medicine goes back even farther in time: all the way back to a village practitioner who lived almost 200 years ago.

Most of my adult life I have tried hard to escape from the gravitational pull of this family history, but mostly I've been unsuccessful. When I think back on it, my struggle to create an individual orbit around medicine (and sometimes to escape from it) began even before I qualified as a doctor from the University of Cape Town in 1967. And in a way, it still continues today.

Growing up in South Africa in such an overwhelmingly medical environment was always a mixed blessing. For one thing, it introduced me early on to an exotic, inverted world – unknown to most people outside it – in which the usually grotesque and shocking all seemed to have become familiar and domesticated. It was the type of world where suffering and death were close acquaintances and not the usual distant strangers, and where the talk around the dinner table, or the barbecue, was often all about Interesting Cases, with their bizarre symptoms, gross swellings, unusual cures or inexplicable deaths.

This background also taught me that medicine is not just about science. It's also all about *stories*, and about the mingling of narratives among doctors, and between them and their patients. As Dr Foster, the general practitioner in Arthur Conan Doyle's story *A Medical Document*, puts it: 'There's no need for fiction in medicine, for the facts will always beat anything you can fancy.' In fact, the art of medicine is a literary art. It requires of the practitioner the ability to listen in a particular way, to empathise and also to imagine – to try to feel what it must be like to be that other person lying in the sickbed, or sitting across the desk from you; to understand the storyteller, as well as the story.

Suburban Shaman is about medicine, and about many of the different types of medical practice. It is written from the perspective of a doctor who is also an anthropologist. It's a view from the inside, from the other side of the doctor's desk, and is based on the 27 years I spent in family practice, before taking early retirement some time ago in order to concentrate on teaching and writing.

This book is not an autobiography. It's a mosaic of memories rather than a single story. It aims to take the reader along on a series of journeys that I've been privileged to make through the various different worlds of doctors and patients – from medical school in South Africa during the darkest days of apartheid, via ship's doctoring in the Mediterranean, to a spell doing research at Harvard Medical School in the USA, to medical aid programmes in the Third World and encounters with shamans and folk healers in different countries, and finally, to the practice of family medicine in various parts of London and surrounding towns. Along the way, each of these different worlds has taught me a specific lesson about the nature of healing and of medical care. Those lessons form the basis of this book.

Much of what follows is a defence of old-style family practice, and a celebration of it. It's a type of medicine that people often take for granted, or even ignore – except when disasters happen. In Britain, the local National Health Service general practitioner or family doctor is still the first point of call for the vast majority of people who seek medical help. In its quiet and unassuming way, and every day of the week, family medicine is still at the very frontline of human suffering.

My own professional life has been spent mainly at this less glamorous end of medicine, in suburban family practice, far from the great fluorescent laboratories of the medical schools and the teaching hospitals, far indeed from the newspaper headlines about the latest wonder drug, or the latest tanned and white-coated celebrity surgeon. Family practice in Britain is a rushed, unglamorous life and the effects of its heavy workload can be grinding and corrosive. Yet, for all of this, I think there's a quiet and unacknowledged heroism about it all. And it may well be one of the last survivors (though not the only one) of a long tradition of 'real' medicine, the type of holistic approach to health care that has always tried to treat the person as well as their disease, and to do this within the context of their own home, their family and their community.

What fascinates me particularly about it are the extraordinary human situations into which people (doctors as well as patients) find themselves propelled by illness, especially sudden, unexpected illness. Medical life provides endless examples of these situations, and they supply some of the tales that follow: brief glimpses through the half-opened doorways of many thousands of lives, revealing moments of drama that are poignant, tragic, bizarre or even comic.

Family practice is a long-term business. Gradually, over time, family doctors need to build up a picture of their patients and their backgrounds: from visiting their homes when they're ill, from treating other members of their families, from consulting their medical records (which follow them from birth, wherever they move), and from seeing them not only in sickness but also in health (for routine examinations, health advice and immunisations). From all of this, they should acquire a deep knowledge of a particular individual and their family. Of course, to achieve this, it helps to be embedded within a particular community, to be a part of its daily life and of its local identity. Although in Britain this type of continuity is much truer of rural rather than urban practice, in the suburbs I have still often encountered my patients in the supermarket or in the street, as well as in the consulting room. Overall, their family doctor is more familiar to them than the white-coated strangers who interrogate and examine them at the local general hospital.

Family practice also involves (or at least, *should* involve) an under-standing of patients' belief systems, the ways they understand how their bodies function, and how they have got ill. And as far as possible, family doctors need to try to work within those beliefs in order to make their interventions most effective. Above all, family practice involves understanding the ways that illness can upset not only a body's inter-nal equilibrium but also the harmony of the patient's relationships with the world they live in – and therefore how treatment should not only treat a diseased organ, but also aim to restore to the patient's life that previous sense of equilibrium.

As well as being a doctor, I have also been trained as an anthropologist. This has given me a certain individual perspective on medical practice, as well as on other systems of healing found elsewhere.

In the early 1970s, I gave up medicine for several years to study social anthropology at London University. I had been wanting to move out of clinical medicine for a while, in order to acquire a fresh perspective on it. Coming from such a medical background, I needed the break.

Anthropologists are people who study many different societies and tribes in depth, and then compare them with one another. They ask questions like: How do they differ from one another? What do they have in common? How do they see their world, and behave within it? Some anthropology graduates, like myself, have also gone on to study the different forms of curing and healing (they're not necessarily the same thing) found in many parts of the world, especially in more traditional societies. There, the questions to be asked include: How do people explain the causes of illness, and other forms of misfortune? Do they blame others for their illness, or themselves? Do they blame germs or spirits, divine punishment or even witchcraft? And to whom do they turn if they do fall ill? A doctor, a priest, a healer? If so, why? Answering these types of questions often involves interviewing traditional folk healers, as I have done in South Africa, Brazil, Europe and elsewhere.

Anthropology gave me the opportunity to learn in some detail about some of the hundreds of different forms of healing found worldwide, many of them flourishing beyond the boundaries of Western medicine, and then to compare and contrast them with our own system of health care: to see modern scientific medicine's many strengths, but also its weaknesses. It led me also to an interest – which I'd never had before – in the traditional African folk healers or shamans back home in South Africa, the *sangomas*, as well as in similar traditional healers elsewhere.

Being both doctor and anthropologist has also given me a different, rather unusual view of the work I was doing (and it's certainly an advantage when working in London, now one of the most multicultural cities on Earth). This double vision has enabled me to observe close up, like some bemused ethnographer, the increasing alienation between the warring 'tribes' of patients and doctors – each with its own specific view of illness, its beliefs about its causes, and expectations of how it should be treated. It has thrown some light on the problems of communication between these two groups, and underlined to me, again and again, the crucial importance of understanding the patient's perspective, as well as the role of family and social context in the shaping of illness, and how it is dealt with. It has also shed light on the two parallel but interconnected forms of health care that exist in Britain – general practice/family medicine on one hand, hospital-based medicine on the other – and to understand the advantages, and disadvantages of each of them.

It took me some time in practice to realise that a fundamental aspect of family medicine was its attitude to uncertainty. After literally tens of thousands of consultations with patients, and many hundreds of house-calls, clinical practice eventually taught me one big, and rather sobering lesson: it's that the more you know about doctoring and why it works (or doesn't work), the more you realise how much you *don't* know. For despite its patina of science, at its core medicine – and not just family medicine – is not really about certainties, nor ever has been. To the disappointment of some of the new breed of 'techno-doctors' as I've called them, it's also about doubt and ambiguity, and ethical dilemmas that are sometimes difficult or even impossible to solve. It's also about the limits of human expertise, especially with serious, chronic or incurable diseases.

Uncertainty is endemic in medicine, and it's the inspiration for much of its research and enquiry. But it's also part of its *frisson* and what makes it such a fascinating, absorbing profession. For, especially in family practice, you never quite know who, or what, will walk through your door next – the diseases they will suffer from, the stories they will tell.

At the level of daily medical practice it means, as the cancer specialist Rachel Naomi Remen puts it: 'Perhaps the most basic skill of the physician is the ability to have comfort with uncertainty, to recognise with humility the uncertainty inherent in all situations, to be open to the ever-present possibility of the surprising, the mysterious, and even the holy, and to meet people there.'

Despite Dr Remen's advice, my own experience is that modern medicine seems to strive increasingly for a world of ultimate certainty. A world devoid of ambiguity, where the wonders of science and technology will provide a clear answer for every human doubt and a clear solution for every human ill; where everything can be measured and everything can be explained, and almost everything can be controlled, even the processes of death and dying. Not surprisingly, one result of this approach is the tendency to see the ill patient's body as just a malfunctioning machine, one that needs merely a mechanical repair, or a new type of chemical fuel, or just the provision of spare parts. A machine that can best be diagnosed, and monitored (and sometimes treated) only by other machines.

But this attempt to reduce much of the complexity of human suffering to a graph or an X-ray plate, a scan or a printout, is doomed to failure. It can never work. It has resulted in many patients perceiving the medical system as becoming even more impersonal and standardised every year. They complain that some doctors concentrate more on the diseased body parts, than on them – the people who contain those body parts. Many say further that it largely ignores their beliefs and fears, their individual needs, feelings and desires. Already the signs of this process of alienation are here: increasing patient dissatisfaction with doctors, more frequent litigation and complaints, media campaigns against the medical profession, and a growing resort to the various forms of 'alternative' medicine.

In the United States, critics of the medical system are even more vocal, seeing it as being in danger of becoming just another industry, a major corporate undertaking in which profits have become more important than people, an industry over-dependent on expensive technology as well as on the pharmaceutical industry. It was something I saw at close range in the mid-1980s, when I spent a year in the USA, teaching and researching (mainly on psychosomatic disorders) at Harvard Medical School That year confirmed to me that for all its wondrous discoveries, modern medicine really was in danger of entering a cul-de-sac, one that could eventually alienate it from many of its patients, and from its traditional tasks of healing as well as of curing.

But even in Britain, with its proud NHS, the impersonal mass-production factory model sometimes seems to have become predominant, with the key aim (or rather 'target') of feeding in the raw material of sick people at one end, and 'producing' larger and larger numbers of healthy people at the other – and all in the shortest possible period of time. This is despite major changes and improvements such as the increase in numbers of women entering medicine, and a greater emphasis on consultation skills. In recent years, too, the case of Dr Shipman, the family doctor who murdered many of his patients, has thrown a dark shadow over the relationships between patients and their doctors.

For many reasons then, family medicine itself seems in danger of moving further away from its original roots, from that well-loved (even if largely mythological) figure of the past – the old-fashioned family doctor with his kindly face and little black bag out visiting the sick on some wintry night, urging on his horse-and-buggy through the blizzards or the driving rain – towards an imitation of hospital medicine. Under the relentless pressures of bureaucracy, cost-effectiveness, rushed consultations, the fear of litigation, the decline in home visits and other factors, those words of Arthur Conan Doyle – 'He goes from house to house', and his step and his voice are loved and welcomed in each. What could a man ask more than that?' – sometimes have a hollow ring about them.

This book was written in answer to two inner imperatives. First, a desire for some resolution within myself of an old (and sometimes painful) split between two different worlds: those of science and art, medicine and literature. And secondly, because of a certain unease and sadness that I feel about some of the directions in which medicine is going. However, despite its occasional polemical tone, I should make absolutely clear that the book is *not* a rejection of scientific medicine. Nor of medical specialisation. Both are necessary, as well as indispensable, but it does make the point that while such specialised skills are necessary, they are not sufficient. Focusing only on a tiny part of the body, but not on the rest – and seeing people only in an impersonal clinic or hospital ward, far removed from their familiar home or family context – is often not enough. Something else is needed.

At medical school, in our textbooks and lectures, diseases were described to us as if they were abstract 'things', somehow independent of the people who suffered from them. And independent, too, of their religious or social backgrounds, or the particular and unique circumstances of their personal lives, such as stress, unhappiness, poverty, discrimination, or poor housing. Most importantly, this approach left out the *meanings* that people give to their illnesses, the sorts questions they ask themselves when they do get ill: 'Why has it happened to *me?*', 'Why *now?*'. It left out, too, all the stories they tell – to themselves and to others – the stories you hear in family practice from across your desk, every day of the week: endless cycles of stories, whether poetic or banal, many hidden within other stories, or concealed behind the masks of symptoms or disease.

Sometimes, in criticising this trend towards the increasingly impersonal approach of high-tech medicine, I sound (even to myself) like a sort of Luddite, someone nostalgic for a mythical, long-lost and low-tech Golden Age of Medicine. Then I have to remind myself, forcefully, that in the 17th century 'nostalgia' was actually the name of a disease, an extreme and pathological form of homesickness. I also have to remember all that medicine has achieved: its great triumphs of surgery and transplantation, the development of new drugs and vaccines, the conquest of many diseases, the decline in infant mortality, the lengthening of the human life-span. Yet despite all of these achievements, I still feel that something is being lost from medicine today, or is in danger of being lost – some precious, elusive quality of human interaction, something invisible and yet at the same time very real.

I have chosen the title *Suburban Shaman* because it seems, to me at least, that some aspects of the work of a family doctor have a distant resemblance to those of a traditional healer. To some this might seem absurd. As a modern doctor one should have absolutely nothing in common with these people, with all their superstitions, their feathers and fur, their strange chants and outlandish rituals. After all, our intellectual roots are completely different – ours in Science, theirs in religion and folk tradition. But I've come to believe from my anthropological studies that different types of healer, whether medical or not, have more in common than might appear – and so do the patients who consult them. After all, under the masks of culture and custom, suffering people want roughly the same things from their healers, in whichever society they happen to live: relief from discomfort, relief from anxiety, a relationship of compassion and care, some explanation of what has gone wrong, and why, and a sense of order or meaning imposed on the apparent chaos of their personal suffering – to help them make sense of it and to cope.

Healers such as the South African *sangoma* are usually dismissed by Western doctors as quacks and charlatans, irrelevant or even dangerous – and many of them undoubtedly are. But with all our science, our sophisticated X-rays, MRI scans and other diagnostic gadgetry, I still think we can learn something from them, just as we can learn from the previous generations of family doctors. It is something that today's rushed, over-specialised, 'techno-doctors' are in danger of forgetting. It's that more holistic view of illness that focuses primarily on a person and not just on their diseased organ; that strives, even if it cannot cure physical disease, then at least to help patients feel better in themselves, more peaceful and more comfortable in their relationships with others, or even with their deities or their natural environment. Such a broader view sees how illness can cause (or result from) an imbalance in a patient's personal cosmos, particularly their connections to those around them, and how, through talk or ritual, social interventions or other treatments, that balance can be restored.

Like previous generations of doctors, what these healers lack in scientific knowledge they often make up for in a shrewd knowledge of human nature, in impressive bedside skills and in a roughly hewn folk wisdom of their own. For all their obvious limitations (and there are many of them) there are some things modern doctors can learn from them, just as the last generations of doctors would have learned lessons from their old horse-and-buggy predecessors. Over the years, I've tried to understand the way they work, the tricks they use. Perhaps most valuable of all, they offer us a window into the past – a glimpse of a more ancient way of healing, now largely replaced by medical science. And it's worth a glimpse, even if the landscape seems at first so unfamiliar.

The sections of the book that follow this Introduction are arranged, more or less, in chronological order: from medical school in South Africa onwards. Along the way, there are some reflections, based on my own experiences – including some mistakes I have made in practice, in both attitude and action – and some clinical tales to illustrate them.

So the question remains. What are the special strengths of modern medicine, and what are its special weaknesses? What, in recent years, has gone wrong with it? And what – if anything – can we learn from other forms of healing found elsewhere in the world?

I offer these tales in the hope that they may go some way towards answering a few of these questions.

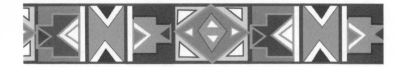

PART
1

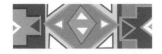

Setting Out

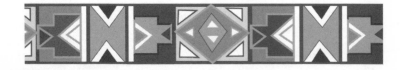

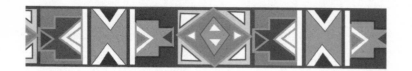

CHAPTER
1

Asylums

It is the 1950s, and I am still at school. My father is an astronaut. Every few years he seems to travel to a different planet. Strange, rectangular planets, usually orbiting through small towns or dusty *dorps*, in the depths of the South African *platteland* or countryside. Actually, he is a government psychiatrist, who works for the oddly named 'Department of Mental Hygiene'. He is a staff psychiatrist and later the head or deputy-head (they call it Physician-Superintendent, or Assistant Physician-Superintendent) of several big psychiatric hospitals, one after the other. These are the planets that I reluctantly land on every year. While all the other children spend their summer holidays on the beach, I spend mine in mental hospitals.

Cradock, Pietermaritzburg, Howick, Krugersdorp, Queenstown, Fort England Hospital in Grahamstown, Weskoppies Hospital outside Pretoria (known locally as *groendakkies* or green roofs). In each place I run barefoot with the other doctors' children, fight and play *bok-bok* and other games with them. In each place I am introduced proudly to every individual member of staff: 'This is my son. He's at school in Johannesburg. He lives there with his mother. He's very artistic. Say hello to Dr Geldenhuys, *boytjie*.'

Driving through the high guarded gates, past the small brick bungalows and coiffured lawns of the senior medical staff, you find yourself entering a different world, a volatile place of unexpected moods and hidden rules. There are some men and women in white coats and white uniforms standing around, others shambling by in pyjamas or dressing gowns, withdrawn, frozen, shouting out or crying, or talking volubly with invisible companions. I am forbidden to speak to them.

Like the asylum at Charenton, in Peter Weiss's play *Marat*, the hospital is to some extent a distorted mirror image of the world outside. By the 1950s, madness is on both sides of the fence. Apartheid is now powerfully pervasive, and my father hates it. By government decree, the Black patients are rigidly segregated from the Whites in his hospital. They sleep in different wards, are given different ('more culturally appropriate') diets, live in different degrees of crowding, and also (though this is seldom spoken of) sometimes given different types of treatment.

One day my father tells me of a rumour about a colleague of his (a psychiatrist, but also the proud possessor of a theology degree), who is said to have given many times the recommended dose of electro-convulsive therapy to his African patients, as part of a post-graduate 'research project'. But no matter, he is supposed to have said, for 'their brains are completely different from our own'. It's odd how soon my memory of this conversation becomes fuzzy, and fades, for no one ever mentions it in my presence again. When I eventually do meet this man, the puzzle deepens. He doesn't look at all like a Dr Mengele. He is plump, amiable, cheerful and bald, a family man, with a kindly face and a booming laugh, probably a stalwart of his local Dutch Reformed Church or even a lay minister. He gives me sweets and slaps me on the back. But is he mad or bad? Is he just living on the wrong side of the asylum fence, or is he evil? Or maybe neither? How could any doctor behave like that? For years of my boyhood I try to puzzle it out. But however I look at it, the sense of unease remains: the apparently unbridgeable gap in my mind between the person I've met and what he's done. For many years it remained as part of my wider South African mystery. A puzzle, without a solution.

Among themselves, my father and his colleagues speak in a peculiar dialect, difficult for any outsider to understand. They speak of strange creatures they refer to as 'psychos' and 'schizos' and 'feebs' (or feeble-minded), sometimes differentiating between 'low-grade feebs' and 'high-grade feebs'. There are bad people called 'psychopaths', people who laugh too much called 'manics', people who don't laugh at all called 'depressives', and some who don't like being laughed at, called 'paranoids'. After many summer holidays, these words become contagious. I find myself beginning to use them on my friends and my relatives, even on myself. Thus, for much of my childhood I come firmly to believe that sadness is the same as depression, mania a type of happiness, 'manic-depression' a combination of the two. And also that being confused is the same as being 'schizoid', while disagreeing too strongly with your parents is the clear sign of a 'psychopath' – bearer of a terrible, yet ill-defined, Mark of Cain.

In the hospital grounds, several 'high-grade feebs' and a heavily-sedated 'schizo' or two water the lawns, or weed the flowerbeds in the garden of my father's bungalow – the one with the white metal burglar-proof bars on the windows, and the large hunting rifle mounted above the fireplace. Part of the peculiar atmosphere of these places comes from the fact that many of them were formerly military camps, their barracks now converted into lengthy wards. Fort Napier Hospital in Pietermaritzburg, for example, where my father worked for several years, was once the base of the British army in Natal from 1843 till 1914, and was especially important to them during the 1879 Zulu War. Later, during the First World War, it was used as an internment camp for German Prisoners-of-War, only becoming a government psychiatric hospital in 1927. It is this atmosphere of high fences, long barracks and straight lines that still signals a place sealed off from everyday life, one where discordant bodies, as well as chaotic emotions, can gradually be brought into line. The atmosphere within it is tense, touchy; the boundaries between 'sanity' and 'madness' only paper thin, though these pieces of paper, once signed and officially stamped, can have very powerful and permanent effects on any individual's life.

At first sight each of these hospitals seems to be an inverted, illogical world, a *mundus inversus*, a world where nothing makes sense. But then, with all the madness of apartheid in full fling outside, you begin to notice a certain quiet peace about them, about their ordered lawns and neat fences, their fixed routines and regular rituals, a certain logical calm. To me, entering and leaving them each summer, they gradually come to seem like a refuge, an asylum.

One year my father invites me to attend a play, in one of his hospitals, acted by the patients themselves. It is late in the afternoon, and the big hall in the hospital grounds is slowly filling up. Outside, in the purple African dusk, the cicadas have already begun to applaud. In the hall, the psychiatrists, the matron and the senior nurses and administrators sit stiffly in the front row, benevolent smiles fixed on their faces. Behind them, sit a row or two of worthy local citizens looking nervously around them. The rest of the audience is made up of nurses, porters, clerical staff, followed by rows of patients – the Whites in front, the Blacks behind. One by one, flushed and excited or vaguely frowning, some twitching all over, they have been slowly guided to their seats by groups of nurses.

When the curtain rises, the atmosphere in the hall suddenly becomes electric. I can feel the row of psychiatrists and senior nurses tense up in their seats beside me. They glance anxiously up at the stage, and then back at the crowd behind them. The stage itself is empty, except for a table, and two wooden chairs. There is a backdrop of a room with a wide-open door leading to a garden, open windows and bright pictures on the wall, all crudely painted on sheets sewn together and rustling in the evening air. The plot of the play is confused, but no one seems to notice. The details are long forgotten – something about jealousy and love, and a missing letter. There is a tall, gangling hero with missing teeth and a guttural Afrikaans accent, a lipsticked heroine with disordered hair, and two or three others in borrowed suits and dresses. They shout out their lines or mumble, occasionally trip or stumble, and throw themselves across the stage in exaggerated leaps. At random, unexpected moments, there is wild, ragged applause from the audience behind us. The air in the hall is charged with suppressed hysteria. My father's hands grip tightly together.

Halfway through the second act, the hero's voice begins to rise alarmingly. He seems disoriented, looking around him with apparent confusion. He is beginning to shout out his lines a little too loudly now.

Even under her sedation, the heroine looks worried. In the aisles, I notice several of the burly male nurses begin to move slowly forward towards the stage. But then suddenly the hero smiles, his voice drops and slurs for a moment, and then he carries on with the script. He makes a joke. Everyone laughs. In the aisles, the nurses relax. After a few more shouted and chaotic dialogues, the curtain falls. Everyone applauds with relief. The psychiatrists and the matron smile at one another, nodding. It has been a great success. The local worthies also look pleased. So this is what the doctors mean by 'drama therapy'. It must be the modern approach to treatment. The patients remain seated as we all file slowly up the aisle and out of the hall, chatting to one another. Outside, in the hot summer African air, the cicadas are still applauding.

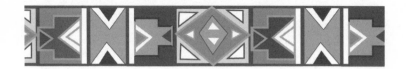

CHAPTER
2

Medical School

We begin simply, climbing our way slowly up the evolutionary tree. First we study a variety of cells and small organisms under the microscope. Then one by one, we dissect worms, snails, cockroaches, dogfish, frogs – almost all the Ten Plagues, in fact, except for the Cape Lobster *Jasus lalandii*, and that token mammal, the white rat. Along the way we are learning the basic medical way of thinking: studying living systems from simple to complex, small to large, part to whole.

After this year of zoology, and other basic sciences, we move on to the study of anatomy and physiology. Every day in the icy dissecting room, there is the exploration of dead, damp grey flesh stinking of preservative. Rows of silent figures swathed in thick plastic sheets, lie in long parallel rows around us. Sometimes it feels to me as though we've wandered into a subterranean tomb filled with ancient mummies. Four of us students – two on each side – dissect our particular cadaver. She is, or rather was, an elderly African woman. We know nothing else about her. We give her a nickname and wonder how she died. We try not to stare at what remains of her genitals. We rest our copies of

Ellis's Anatomy, with its greasy annotated pages, on top of her face or her opened chest cage. The other two students are much keener than we are. Their half of the body is being dismantled at a much faster rate than ours, the sodden muscles, veins and nerves coming into view long before our half does. Perhaps they are cleverer than us in other ways too. For soon their side looks less human every day, resembling even closer the illustrations printed in our anatomy textbooks. Years later, the two of them become physicians specialising in only tiny parts of the body, while on our slow side we both become family doctors.

Before we dissect the cadavers, our tutors inject red dye into the arteries, blue dye into the veins. They strive to make them resemble, as closely as possible, the bright illustrations in our anatomy textbooks. In all this, we are learning an important lesson of medical education – how to turn death into an artefact, an abstract idea or even a form of art. Using our scalpels, we are gradually turning the human body into a piece of art – a three-dimensional textbook, a sculpture of itself, a *Gray's Anatomy* spread out before us. In the dissecting room it seems to me that Nature is being made to imitate Art, for only in this way can the fear of death be kept at bay.

In resonance with the South African world outside the medical school, we are also imposing with our scalpels a type of apartheid on the body – a splitting of the whole into named parts. It's the way that anatomy is taught, but in dismantling the human image we are also in a way dismantling ourselves. Something else is in danger of dying in the dissecting room: a unified sense of what is human, an ancient shape in the mind.

The study of physiology is fascinating – the way the body actually works, the subtle way that it's been organised to move and to metabolise, to feed and renew itself, to create energy from its diet, to adjust to so many different environments, both inside itself and out. One doesn't have to be religious to see it all as a miracle of design or to wonder at the way that muscles contract; that nerves transmit their impulses, smoothly and with little interruption; the ways that the endocrine glands secrete and control their hormones, in a series of delicate feed-back loops, to maintain an inner homeostasis. It all seems to make sense, in a marvellous and logical way. And all this internal bustle and activity, all these rushing blood cells and circulating hormones, these pulsing systoles and complex metabolic cycles, are a welcome antidote to the dead, still, stinking silence of the dissecting room.

After the traumas of dissection and exams, we move on to the third year, with its more detailed studies of actual diseases. Now there is a new affliction. 'Medical student's disease', a well-known form of hypochondria, afflicts many of the class. Studying one grisly disease after another, many of us develop the 'typical' profile of its symptoms and physical signs. With horror, we realise that the disease is no longer distant: it has jumped off the page and entered into our bodies. And we are now *it*, the illustrations in our own medical textbooks. It is terrifying. Soon I am one of those trekking off regularly to the X-ray department or going surreptitiously to the lab for a blood test or two. But that year, Nature really does imitate Art, and in a tragic way. During our lectures on the ear and its many diseases, particularly on a rare tumour called an acoustic neuroma, several students develop, predictably, its 'typical' buzzing in the ears and loss of hearing. One by one, they go off for tests and reassurance. Only this year, things are different. For one particular student, unfortunately, the tests prove not to be negative.

It's difficult to avoid the ubiquity of death. Even my room in the student residence overlooks the mortuary, with its tall belching chimney and the small post-mortem room next door. Just behind it is an old cemetery, and in the far distance the blue-green hills of Milnerton, where a friend and I go horse-riding on most Sunday mornings. Several times a day, just below my window, an unmarked blue van drives down from the big hospital up on the hill. Then there is the clanking of doors, and another white-swathed figure is wheeled out on a trolley and into the building like an ancient mummy. And each time, when the tall chimney belches a while later, a sweet, sickly, unsettling smell drifts along the corridors of the student residence, and creeps into our rooms and between the pages of our textbooks – and then eventually into our dreams.

Death by day, art by night. In the evenings, to deal with the morbid events of the day, I decide to take life drawing classes. I have always drawn, even from infancy, encouraged by my mother, who herself had graduated in 1937 from the University of Cape Town's Michaelis School of Fine Art. The classes are held in the early evenings at an art school on Green Point Common, an old colonial building, and the big room crowded with easels is filled with a cool sea breeze and the smell of ozone from the Atlantic coast only a few hundred yards away. Here for several hours, I can contemplate pink, naked flesh – untouchable, but at least alive – instead of the grey, damp, icy flesh of the day, with its sour stink of formaldehyde. Twice a week, using charcoal or pencil, I can create new life on every blank page. It's the only way I can cope.

Studying physiology – and from the fourth year onwards, clinical medicine and surgery – is also, in an indirect way, a literary experience: for there's a certain poetry in the actual words that are used, the technical terms that our lecturers give to different diseases, organ processes or even symptoms. These exotic, unfamiliar, alliterative words remain in one's mind many years after medical school as a sort of archaic and mysterious poetry: 'dysdiadochokinesia' (a neurological symptom), 'whispering pectoriloquy' (a distinctive sound, heard through the stethoscope), 'angioneurotic oedema' (an allergic swelling of the body), 'hydatidiform mole' (a type of growth in the uterus), 'thyrotoxicosis' (over-activity of the thyroid gland), and 'sternocleido-mastoideus' (a muscle in the neck). Even the word 'anti-biotic' has a puzzling ring to it. What are those 'biotics' that everyone is so against?

Physiology and anatomy, in particular, also provide a rich set of metaphors that everyone – not only doctors – uses on a daily basis. The media speak fluently of the 'head' of a government, the 'heart' or 'lifeblood' of a community, the 'brains' behind a conspiracy, the way that some events are 'difficult to digest'. Monosyllabic words for the genitals, or for sex or excretion, pepper everyday conversation. The subject of Immunology, especially, has provided much of the language that is still woven into the discourse on immigration, the language of xenophobia, in which immigrants and refugees are referred to as if they were 'foreign bodies', 'transplanted' from one country to another – and who in the new place encounter a range of 'host-reactions': from 'acquired tolerance' and 'hypersensitivity' to outright 'rejection', often followed by a violent assault on them by 'anti-bodies' and even 'killer cells'. It's tough to be a 'foreign body' – whether in the body or out there in society.

Cape Town Medical School has the usual Cast of Characters. The ones you find at almost every medical school. There are the jocks and the rugger-buggers, swilling their cans of Castle Lager, and always training for the next big match; the boisterous party people, cheerful and bleary eyed every Monday morning, opening their textbooks only a few nights before their exams; the clumps of swots and nerds, bespectacled, intense, their systematic study plans tacked neatly to the walls above their desks (future professors of medicine, surgery, or anything else); the bearded old-young men, puffing away at their pipes, and muttering gravely about *angst* and existentialism (future psychiatrists, many of them); the religious ones, with pale faces and rimless glasses, a Bible on one side of their desk, a pile of textbooks on the other; the intense young women with beehive hair-do's and deep, Lillian Gish mascara, pulling mournfully on their long cigarettes, their rooms filled with the paperbacks of Virginia Wolf and Simone de Beauvoir, with jazz and Joan Baez. And then there are the silent majority of us – white-coated, rushing, worrying, partying, drinking, studying, and then studying some more – future general practitioners, dermatologists, paediatricians, pathologists and all the rest.

Among a tiny but vocal minority of students, racism is rife. The colonialists from Up North are the very worst. One day in 1964 we are sitting in someone's room in the student residence, a whole crowd of us. It's a historic day further north in Africa, for Northern Rhodesia has just become independent of Britain. Now it's called the Republic of Zambia, with Dr Kenneth Kaunda as its first President. One of the students from up there is Tom, and now his florid face is contorted with wonder and contempt as he sneers at the *munts* who have taken over 'my country'. He uses the word again and again, a derogatory term for Africans, much used by white colonialists in Rhodesia and elsewhere. 'What a bunch of *munts*,' he says, 'what a bunch of *munts*!'

Tom passes round a small pamphlet about the new Republic that he's just been sent as a Zambian studying abroad. It is full of facts and figures about the new country, brightly illustrated, as well as a tiny Zambian flag. He points to the coloured photograph of President Kaunda on the back cover, dressed in an elaborate uniform, with epaulettes, gold buttons and gold braid. 'Isn't that so typical of a *munt*,' he says, shaking his head, ' to make himself a fancy, crazy uniform like that. Isn't that just typical of them!' No one says anything in the room, but the pamphlet passes around. Suddenly, someone pipes up: 'Hold on a sec, Tom,' he says, 'You didn't read the caption under the photo'. He reads out what it says: Kaunda is wearing the uniform of an Honorary Colonel of one of the elite regiments of the British Army, one of the regiments, I think, that guard the Queen. It's not an African uniform at all! For a moment, Tom looks ashen, confused. There is silence in the room. Everyone is looking at him now, wondering how he will extricate himself.

'Well,' he says, after a long, long pause, 'trust a *munt* to *wear* a uniform like that!'

The Cape summers are warm and sensual. Clifton Beach (in those days a 'Whites Only' beach) waits for me every weekend, the Atlantic surf exploding wildly on the rocks offshore, the sand covered with acres of oiled bodies tanning in bright bikini's, rotating themselves slowly from one side to the other like kebabs in the sun. Back in the laboratory we watch starfish sperm fertilise starfish ova, the cells mingling in silent, romantic ecstasy on a tiny microscope slide. I dream of dead bodies, and also of live ones. There are lots of parties, but not much action. Sex, like democracy, seems almost illegal in our country. Television has been forbidden in South Africa (the Dutch Reformed Church disapproves of it), and there are no girlie magazines to be found. So what else is a young man to do, but peek surreptitiously at page 1406 of *Gray's Anatomy*, the one with the big engraving of 'The Female External Genitalia'. 'The female organ of copulation,' it says, 'is a fibromuscular tube lined with stratified epithelium.' A fibromuscular tube! A moist mysterious opening of language and of flesh. The page is soon wrinkled from constant reading. A fibromuscular tube! To me those words sound like Latin poetry, a Tantric rhyme.

In 1967, the year of our final examinations, we are the excited but distant witnesses of one of the greatest landmarks of medical history: the first ever human heart transplant, carried out by Dr Christiaan Barnard, one of our professors. Before the operation, many of us had seen the recipient in the ward, and some had even examined him. All of a sudden, Groote Schuur Hospital is at the centre of world attention. In all this fuss and excitement, I am in awe not only of the technical brilliance of the operation, but also of its symbolic importance. The operation teaches me the enormous power of language, for the surgeon has strayed into a landscape of metaphors, where the 'heart' is seen not just as a muscular pump, but also as a universal symbol for emotion, courage, intimacy and will.

For one of the first times in human history, language and flesh have come together. At the moment that the borders of one body have been breached by the symbolic core of another, the protective barriers between Nature and Art – between physical reality and the language we use to signify it – are suddenly dissolved. Never again will phrases like 'sick at heart', 'heartless', 'to give heart' or 'to take heart' have quite the same meaning to me. In a miracle of medical science, donor and recipient have, quite literally, 'lost their hearts' to one another, through the agency of the matchmakers of medical science, so that one can be as 'hearty' as before. Somehow, my image of the human body will never be quite the same again.

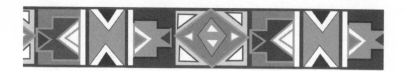

CHAPTER
3

Side-Show

It is an early summer's day. Walking along the polished linoleum floor of one of the 'Whites Only' medical wards, between neat rows of starched beds, I find myself at the fourth bed on the left. It is the bed of the man whom I, as a first-year clinical student new to the wards, have been assigned to 'clerk': to question, examine, diagnose, prognosticate, and then report on to my tutors. This is an essential part of our training, and yet now I stand at the allocated bedside and blink. And then blink again. It seems to me like an optical illusion, or a hallucination. It surely must be. The man in the hospital bed simply cannot be there.

It is Cape Town in the 1960s. The whole country is a brittle place, tense and besieged. Beginning in 1948 with the unexpected election victory of the Afrikaner Nationalists, its entire multi-coloured population has been legally dissected by the laws of apartheid, as if by the scalpel of some demented anatomist. A law called the Population Registration Act of 1950 has cut up the population into two huge slices, called 'Whites' and 'Non-Whites'. And then into smaller pieces: Europeans, Africans, Coloureds, Asians, Chinese, with multiple subdivisions of these as well. The harsh laws of 'separate development' as they call it, have cut communities by colour, sliced them apart by language, territory or tribe.

By the time I enter medical school in 1962, all the suburbs and schools in the country have been rigidly divided. So have the churches, restaurants, banks, bars, hospitals, beaches, post offices, public toilets, park benches and railway stations, cemeteries and swimming pools. Segregation is total, marked always by signs reading *Whites Only/Slegs Blankes*, and sometimes by high brick walls, barbed wire and the snarl of guard dogs. Members of the different communities are forbidden by law to live together, play together, love together, even die together. The country is now a pigmentocracy, in which the 'Non-Whites' will always be second-class citizens.

Like all the others, Groote Schuur Hospital, our own teaching hospital in Cape Town, has been surgically bisected. Now it consists of two adjoining wings: one for 'White' patients, the other for 'Non-Whites'. At a few of the nursing stations in the wards, there stands a holder for thermometers, two long tubes of disinfectant clamped to a board and clearly labelled 'White Oral' and 'White Rectal', while on the other side of the building they read 'Non-White Oral' and 'Non-White Rectal'. A friend of mine, bearded and intense, sees himself as a radical *agent provocateur*. He delights (when no-one is watching) in switching the thermometers around. Winking wildly at this major revolutionary act, he is convinced of the mortal damage that will be done to apartheid by a particular thermometer, once jammed up a black rectum, now being inserted into a lily-white mouth. (Thirty years later when apartheid finally *does* collapse – surprisingly, with more of a whimper than a bang – I recall his conspiratorial nudges. Can he somehow take credit for it all? For having released a tiny wave of absurd juxtapositions, a cascade of synchronicity and interlinked events that grew and grew, swelling into the mighty wave that finally swept it all away?).

Within the medical school, government decrees have forbidden the Non-White medical students from ever examining white patients, barring them from the inflammatory sight of naked white flesh, whether alive or dead. They are even forced to dissect their Non-White cadavers far away from the rest of us, clustered together at one fluorescent-lit end of the long, icy dissecting room.

In 1966, only a few miles away from the medical school, one of the most notorious examples of apartheid 'ethnic cleansing' is taking place: the total destruction of District Six. It's an area of only about one square mile, just near the centre of town, but it's been racially 'mixed' for centuries. In its heyday, District Six was like a miniature Lower East Side or London's East End, right at the tip of Africa – a vibrant, chaotic melting-pot of colour and class, race and religion, its population Christian, Jewish, Muslim and Hindu. In colour its occupants are white, yellow, black, brown and many interesting shades in-between – in short, an apartheid bureaucrat's worst nightmare. It is a poor area, but it's still the single most multiracial spot in all of southern Africa, a tiny precognition of Nelson Mandela's 'Rainbow Nation'.

In 1966 this mixed history is being brought to an end, with the brutal expulsion of its entire Coloured population of 55,000 people, followed by the destruction of the District itself, house by house. The inhabitants are being sent to windy, flea-bitten 'Coloured Group Areas' on the Cape Flats, many miles out of town. Even a decade after the end of apartheid, Cape Town will still be suffering from the psychic and social wounds of this event: crime, poverty, family breakdown, and the rest. But in the 1960s, except for the occasional protest march, petition or candlelit vigil, it doesn't really affect our busy, book-lined medical student lives. Exams still come and go. Senator Robert Kennedy visits the campus from America and gives us a rousing anti-apartheid speech. Everyone cheers. There are more exams. One of the medical students commits suicide; others drop out with exhaustion.

I open my eyes again. And the man in the bed is still there. So is the ward itself, with all its pungent and familiar odours, that complex collage of flowers and floor polish, of linoleum, pus and disinfectant. And the view out of the big windows is still the same: the small higgledy-piggledy houses of the suburb of Observatory on one side, the slopes of Devil's Peak on the other.

I look at the man again. Emerging from an oversized pair of blue-striped pyjamas is a dark neck, and an even darker face, and two dusky hands that nervously clasp and unclasp each other on top of the white starched sheets. In a 'Whites Only' ward, a Coloured man lies in the bed!

He is in his late fifties with a bald head, drooping features, a prominent upper lip, and an unusual greyish-brown coloration to his skin and the folds of his face – almost as if they were permanently in shadow. He looks up at me warily as I stand at the foot of his bed, and I introduce myself.

Mr Pritchard is a former warehouse manager in a big factory outside of town. He has an unfamiliar accent. In fact, it turns out he is not South African at all, but an immigrant from England – from Yorkshire, I think.

In my new white coat with its prominent green plastic name-tag and the green stripe around the sleeves, I like to see myself, at last, as a real doctor. Like the other clinical students, I glance surreptitiously downwards at regular intervals, checking that my stethoscope still pokes prominently out of my side-pocket. Then I take out my notepad, set it on my knees and look up at him, trying with difficulty to assemble my features into a professional mask of informed compassion. Just like a *real* doctor.

Over the next half an hour or so, I take a full medical 'history', making copious notes of his story. But it soon becomes clear Mr Pritchard is actually the bearer of two very different tales, two different histories. And only one of these could ever be found within the pages of my medical textbooks.

Slowly, frowning often and taking frequent sips of orange squash from the table besides him, he describes how, many months before, he had developed overwhelming symptoms of bodily fatigue, a peculiar lack of energy that had got worse every day, until at last he hardly had the strength to get through the day. Then there was nausea, and often he was sick. Sometimes he also had diarrhoea. And then quite slowly, almost imperceptibly, he began to notice something else about his body – slow, subtle changes of his skin which filled him with bewilderment, then with horror.

He holds up his dark hands for me to see, palms up, then palms down. He rolls up his sleeves. He points at his face. He points at his feet.

'You see what has happened,' he says, 'You see! I could hardly believe it then – and I can hardly believe it now.'

He gives me a wry, irregular smile.

'But now I'll show you something really funny. Here, young man, look at this.' He unbuttons his pyjama jacket. I lean forward. Under the greying chest hair, the skin is hardly pigmented. In fact, it's really white.

I finish my examination and stand up to go. I look at my watch. But now he is gripping me by the sleeve of my new white coat. 'Please don't go', he says, 'Look, there's something else I want to show you. Please. Just before you go, have a look at all this. '

He sits up slowly and, leaning unsteadily sideways, fumbles inside the white metal locker besides his bed, searching among toothpaste and soap, a copy of yesterday's *Cape Argus* and several bottles of guava juice.

He takes out a thick pile of papers, tied with string, and lays them out before me, one by one, across the coarse hospital blanket. Then shuffles them, as if they were a deck of tarot cards that might somehow foretell a different fate. First he points to a sheaf of family photographs taken many years ago, his dark index finger returning, again and again, to the same small pale face of a young boy in each of the photographs. Then there's his big British birth certificate, creased, folded and torn; his hospital card; the folded green card of his driving licence (and here that same dark finger hovers briefly over his address in a White, working-class suburb); his membership card of a local sports club; his army discharge papers; several letters from his family doctor testifying to his condition, and one or two from his employer. And finally, most potent talisman of all, the small green plastic rectangle of his identity card. For emblazoned clearly in red across it, in Afrikaans and in English, are the three most powerful words of those times: '*Blanke – White Person*'. He smiles a secret, private smile.

Then he lifts up his hands again and stares at them, palms up, then palms down. He shakes his head.

'My God,' he says, and shrugs, 'Can you believe it? What's happened to me? Here, have another look.'

Again he picks up the documents from the bed, and again he hands them over to me, staring closely at my face. He's stopped smiling. Most of the other students have already finished 'clerking' their patients and left the ward. It is quiet now, almost dusk. At the other end of the ward, the nurses are preparing the evening medications. You can just hear the first faint rattles of the dinner trolleys being wheeled along the corridor.

He still won't let me leave. He draws a deep, whistling breath and shakes his head, as if to expel something from it. His voice is husky now. He sips some more orange squash. He explains how he's almost gone hoarse from explaining, day after day, the same story.

'No, I'm *not* a Non-White – and I'm *not* an Indian, either. Really, I'm a White man, a European, just like you.'

He had explained it to everyone he met – to the bus conductor on the Whites Only bus; to the clerk in the segregated post-office, the ticket-seller in the local 'bioscope' or cinema; to all those big, glaring policemen who approach him, day after day; to neighbours and to his friends; even to his family. Every day he has to explain again. 'It must be some sort of suntan,' a friend joked, 'but it's sure lasted a very long time!'

As his skin darkens into the shadows of late afternoon, so does the packet of documents seem to expand. He had carried it around in his inner pocket, where it eventually seemed to harden into a heavy rectangular tumour that began to drag him down like a stone. But after a while, these paper talismans no longer protected him. He describes to me the fateful windy afternoon when, despite his protests, he was thrown out of the Whites-Only carriage of a suburban commuter train ('*Voetsak*! Get out of here! What the hell do you think you're doing in here?'). And the catcalls a few days later at a municipal swimming pool. And then a certain ugly incident in a barber's shop and another on a bus into town – not to mention the unpleasant scene in a suburban restaurant when the police were actually called.

Gradually, he stopped explaining to people. He withdrew from ordinary social life: from the beach and the bar, the bioscope and the *braaivleis*. His employers laid him off, with vague promises of re-employment 'when you feel a bit better'. One by one his friends fell away, with mumbles of embarrassment. Over the many months, he and his wife withdrew even further – huddling at home behind drawn curtains, afraid to venture out together into the streets of Cape Town, for fear of arrest as a racially 'mixed' (and therefore illegal) couple in terms of the government's 1950 Immorality Act.

Several days later, the solution to Mr Pritchard's diagnostic mystery becomes clear, at least, on the physical level. For blood tests and X-rays and various other investigations all confirm what has long been suspected, that he has Addison's Disease. It's one of rarest hormonal disorders and results from the failure of the cortex (or outer part) of the adrenal glands, two small but vital organs that perch atop each of the kidneys. Among many other hormones, they produce 'cortisol' – a hormone crucial for the functioning of the human body. If its level is insufficient in the blood, then there is often an increasing pigmentation of certain parts of the body, especially those not covered by clothing: the face, the neck, the interior of the mouth, the arms and legs, the hands and feet.

Over the next few days a curious, almost electrical atmosphere develops in the ward, with Pritchard's bed at its centre. It feels to me like one of those dark congested moods, that damp heaviness of the air that you sometimes find in the African veldt, just before the violent burst of a thunderstorm. For every day a corona of whispers and suppressed hysteria surrounds him on all sides. Standing at his bedside, I glance around me at the sideways smiles of the other patients, the awkward clumps of medical students that linger about us.

'Hey, there's a white man in the ward -' someone giggles, behind his hand '- *who's turned into a Black*!'.

And it's almost the same thing, a day or so later, when he is presented – as one of a number of 'Interesting Cases' – to serried rows of white-coated doctors and medical students, packed into a large semi-circular lecture theatre elsewhere in the building. It's difficult to forget the look on that dusky, terrified face as he sits hunched in his bathrobe in the middle of this tableau, illuminated under a fluorescent sky, searching the auditorium vainly for a familiar face, his hands nervously clasping and unclasping as eminent physicians drone on and on about him.

I have never seen anything like this before, nor felt such an atmosphere, and yet at the same time there is something very familiar about it. After a while I realise what it reminds me of – the description I'd once read in a book about P.T. Barnum and that great 19th century showman's famous 'Freak Shows' (often the 'side-show' to his travelling circus 'The Greatest Show on Earth'), that for decades were a popular form of entertainment in the USA and elsewhere. For on display in the gaudy, crowded tents of 'P.T. Barnum's Great Travelling Museum, Menagerie, Caravan and Hippodrome' you could see what he claimed were the Tallest, Thinnest, Fattest, Tiniest, Hairiest, Strongest, Ugliest and Oddest people alive. Standing awkwardly on roped-off pedestals, or arranged in *tableaux vivant* as huge crowds milled around them, gawking and sniggering, were what Barnum called 'Wonders of Nature', 'Living Human Prodigies", or even 'Old Dame Nature's Animated Jokes'.

It's significant that, like Mr Pritchard, many of these 'exhibits' also suffered from hormonal disorders – from too much, or too little, of one of those secret alchemical substances that circulate in every human bloodstream. Even today, it's not too difficult for any sharp-eyed doctor who looks closely enough at Barnum's garish posters or photographs of the time to spot the hypopituitariism of Tiny Tim or the Midget Man, the hyperpituitary gigantism of the Giant Giantess or the Tallest Man in the World, the adrenogenital syndrome of the Bearded Lady, the broad hands and coarse physiognomy of the strong man with acromegaly. And familiar, too, is the peculiar expression on many of their faces, as they pose in tableaux for the camera – that curious amalgam of embarrassment and pride.

It is not long after our first meeting – only a few weeks, I think – that Mr Pritchard's 'history' comes to a sudden end. One night he dies silent and solitary in the ward. To most of us, it is not unexpected. I imagine that they buried him in the Whites-Only section of the cemetery after all, and maybe his fat packet of documents with him.

Many years later, I still find myself thinking of him. For people like him, Dr Eric J. Cassell's remark that 'doctors do not treat diseases, they treat people who have diseases' is true, of course, but it is also never quite enough. Beyond the disease is the person, but beyond the person are always the time and place and particular circumstances in which they live and die.

To me Mr Pritchard's predicament illustrates, above all, that diseases never live alone. You cannot ever consider them – as most medical textbooks still do – as independent 'things', entities that somehow float free of the unique realities of a human life. For Mr Pritchard in South Africa of the 1960s, cortisol and apartheid proved to be deadly twins, a fatal combination. Less than a century after P.T. Barnum's death, the fall of that one particular hormone in Mr Pritchard's bloodstream had propelled him unwillingly into a parallel world. He had become his double, his dusky *doppelganger*.

The Darkest Man in the Ward.

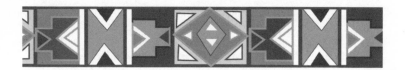

CHAPTER
4

Casualties

It's Friday night in the Casualty Department of Groote Schuur Hospital in Cape Town. It's the mid-1960s and, in our new white coats with green stripes on our sleeves, I and the other medical students are helping out, getting experience. In the factories and small businesses of Cape Town, Friday is always payday, and while some workers make the best of their temporary affluence, others try to relieve them of it. It is the night when the Devil asks his due.

Ten o'clock, and the Casualty Department is already a screaming war zone of split lips and dangling earlobes, swollen eyes and smashed limbs, of blood drip-drip-dripping onto the linoleum floor. Nurses, doctors and medical students – and often policemen – are running here and there, quickly injecting, suturing, resuscitating, attending to one victim, before being called frantically to another. There are shouts and whimpers, the clank of instruments, the purr of the monitor machines, and in the background the banshee wail of distant sirens. One by one, or sometimes in groups of two or three, the victims are brought in by ambulance, taxi or police van. They have stab wounds or fractured skulls, smashed-in ribcages or bloodied limbs that dangle from shreds of flesh. Tonight there has been a gang fight, a domestic shooting, and a collision between a car and a truck packed full of workers on their way home to the townships.

Many of the casualties come from the other Cape Town, the invisible one which most of us know little about, the one on the other side of the mirror: the chaotic slums and shanty towns out on the windy Cape Flats, with their African and Coloured inhabitants. It's a world of raw sewage and leaking roofs, of draughty walls and sudden fires, of knives and beer and over-crowded hopelessness – all the detritus of people dumped there by apartheid, with its resultant poverty and chaos. This is the Cape Town the tourists never see, and which – even though they pass it on the way from the airport – somehow still lies just beyond their imagination. It's a world parallel to the beautiful little city under brooding Table Mountain, with its avenues of historic oaks, its big hotels, long beaches, whitewashed colonial houses, and mostly affluent white population.

Friday night is when all those sculptors of human flesh – the maestros of the knife, the broken bottle, and the sharpened bicycle spoke – show their skills. Occasionally, the police drag one of them into Casualty, shouting and vomiting, and handcuff him to a blood-stained gurney. There he lies, tattooed and toothless, pants half hanging off his buttocks, drunk on cheap wine and *dagga*, his body decorated haphazardly with knife slashes or bullet wounds. It's difficult to imagine that men like that were once someone's child, a loved, cooing, cuddled baby. Now they lie amid the sour smells of vomit and beer, draped on gurneys and trolleys, oozing blood and urine. Hieronymus Bosch would feel quite at home here, on the other side of the mirror, the side that reflects nothing back, only dumb despair.

Lying among the other casualties tonight is a young woman, a student, who has taken an overdose of pain-killing tablets. In a slurred voice, she tells the medical student who first interviews her that it's all because of love – too little, or too much, I forget. Either way, she lies now in the middle of all this noisy chaos, dozy and confused, her dress riding high up her thighs, while two nurses jam a thick rubber tube into her mouth, and then down to her stomach, in order to 'wash it out'. They are angry and impatient. Their movements are rough and merciless. Despite her faint groans that 'It's all his fault,' you can hear them muttering about her to each other about how she has done this to herself, made herself ill. Haven't they got more important things to do with their time, especially on a Friday night? Once more, and with renewed rage, they jam the tube firmly down her gagging throat.

Another Friday night, and in another hospital, just outside Cape Town. It is almost midnight, when suddenly the swing doors burst open, and a woman on a trolley is wheeled in by paramedics, with a crowd of policemen running in behind them. Then another trolley comes in, this time with a man on it, shouting out in Afrikaans, his voice slurred. It is not clear at first, which one of them is the victim. Both smell heavily of whisky and wine. Both are what are called 'Poor Whites' – poor and unskilled yet, in terms of the apartheid laws of the time, part of a privileged aristocracy compared with the Blacks.

The police wheel the man into a nearby cubicle, where he lies in his stained grey trousers and torn T-shirt, shouting, sobbing and threshing about. A policeman takes up position next to him.

'Man, if she dies in there, ' he says to me, 'then this bloke here…' . He doesn't finish, only passes his fingers across his neck, with a quick hissing sound.

Meanwhile, back in the main emergency area, they have cut open her blouse to have a look. Just below her left clavicle, there is a tiny hole, oozing blood, a thin trickle of blood. Someone says she'd been shot during a drunken row, a row that went too far. It must have been a small-calibre gun, for the hole is very small. The woman is still screaming a drunken jumble of obscenities. What is she saying? We insert an intravenous drip into her arm, give her oxygen, call frantically for tests and blood transfusions and the mobile X-ray machines. Nurses scream into telephones, other doctors are called. But then suddenly, quite abruptly, she begins to slow down. She begins to move now only in slow-motion, and her voice, too, becomes slower and slower, her shouts increasingly blurred and indistinct. Suddenly she is silent and falls back heavily onto the trolley as if someone, somewhere, has just unplugged her power supply. Now there are alarms, bleepers, loud shouting and the blur of movement. Nurses, doctors, porters rush around. A thoracic surgeon and then an anaesthetist run breathlessly into Casualty. Together with them, we run her trolley into the elevator, straight up to the operating theatre on the next floor.

A crowd of oxygen cylinders, tubes, monitor machines, bottles of blood and the glinting clatter of silver instruments, suddenly appear around us. Without an anaesthetic, without masks or proper gowns, the surgeon and his assistant cut frantically into her rib cage, searching for the source of her bleeding to clamp it, repair it, before the internal haemorrhage goes too far. The surgeon searches inside her chest, moving organs and vessels aside, his instruments soon lost in a whirlpool of blood. Without his protective mask, I can see how the expression on his face changes abruptly. The reason for this soon becomes clear, for the bullet has nicked a major artery and blood is gushing out of the spreading hole, faster than he can possibly patch it. It is pumping out still, but slower now and weaker. A few moments later and suddenly the surgeon stops, shakes his head and angrily throws down his blood-stained instruments. He peels off his rubber gloves, glances carefully up at the clock on the wall. No one meets his eye as he walks quickly out of the room.

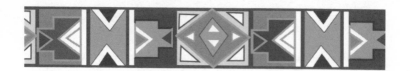

CHAPTER 5

The Green Mask

I sometimes think that there is something about wearing a mask that touches on the numinous, the intangible – even a surgical mask. Masks somehow free you to become someone else, someone much larger than yourself. You feel less constrained, but also *different*. For a moment your old identity disappears, and you can easily take on another; one long hidden, perhaps, deep within yourself. You can become brave and bold, or outrageously sexual. You can become like a character out of a carnival or from the *commedia dell'arte*, or one of the masked Superheroes of comic-book mythology: Captain Marvel, Batman, Spiderman or the Lone Ranger. You can become a masked wrestler, or a bandit like Dick Turpin or Jesse James. You can become a hero – or a villain. If you're a medical student, you can even imagine yourself as a *real* surgeon. The first time I ever put on one of those green surgical masks, I remember how it gave me a curious feeling of unexpected power, of suddenly being able to see things` and do things that I could never have done before.

It was only several years later, studying anthropology in London, that I came across Mircea Eliade's famous essay on tribal masks and his description of how, in many such societies, these masks are not just artistic objects. They are also all about *transformation*. For in certain ceremonies of the tribe they are the means of a mystical metamorphosis of ordinary human beings into animals or birds, heroes or ancestors, spirits or gods. In some Native American tribes of the Pacific North-West, for example, the masked dancers in their annual rituals believe that they actually become the Bears, Wolves, Ravens or Eagles whose masks they wear. In each case these masks enable the wearer to cross, temporarily, the invisible line that divides the ordinary world from the world of the supernatural. It's a phenomenon that's been reported by anthropologists from many parts of the world. In their sacred winter ceremonies, tribes like the Kwakiutl act out their possession and 'devouring' by special bird or animal spirits, portrayed by other masked dancers – such as Cannibal Raven or Cannibal Grizzly Bear. For Eliade, such masks also affect one's perception of time, in that 'the time implied by the mask is ecstatic time, removed from the here and now.' All masks used in ritual, he says, give the wearer that curious sense of timelessness, of a numinous time, free of the usual constraints of the calendar and the clock. They transform the wearer back to what he calls 'primordial mythological time' – a form of time that can only be lived by becoming the mystical 'other'.

Although surgical masks are worn solely for a practical purpose – to reduce the threat of infection to the patient – I believe they may also have another, more subliminal role. To my anthropological eye it seems that, in addition to the merely technical procedure, something else is going on during a surgical operation, something rather akin to those tribal ceremonies. For with their fixed rituals and choreography, their standardised costumes, and rigid rules of behaviour and speech, surgical operations can also be seen as a type of masque, an allegorical performance carried out by masked actors. In this setting, the mask helps transform an ordinary mortal doctor into a type of archetypal superhero, someone daring and brave. In this cool green, disinfected operating 'theatre', with its beeping machines and low murmuring voices, this masked hero is now ready to confront the forces of Disease and Death – and defeat them; to impose, with the help of all the powers of Science that he incarnates, Order onto Chaos. And in doing so, he breaks one of the greatest taboos of all: the invasion, and dismantling, of a living human body. For the surgeon is the only person in our society allowed to slash open a living body in order to repair it, to heal one wound by creating another.

In her studies of American surgeons, the anthropologist Joan Cassell has described them as a predominately masculine society, one that 'admires cars, sports, speed, competence'. She sees similarities between their world and those of other modern superheroes, such as test pilots and astronauts. Like them 'the successful surgeon takes risks, defies death, comes close to the edge, and carries it off'. Her surgeons see themselves as being 'invulnerable, untiring, unafraid of death or disaster'. Each one is 'a macho, martial hero who combats disease and rescues patients from death'. 'You couldn't have a good surgeon who didn't believe in the concept of the Hero,' says one Chief of a Department of Surgery to her, for each surgical intern worth his salt 'would like to be a hero.' 'You have to approach an operation like a battle', says another. To the *American Medical Association News* of 1982 the surgeon 'above all else is a soldier,' and 'this healer greets every day as a battle'.

Most of the surgeons Joan Cassell meets are self-confident, swash-buckling men of action, decisive and daring. Many seem to like taking risks, at least in their off-duty lives: some even refuse to use their car seat-belts while driving, others use them only reluctantly. Some are proud of not wearing overcoats, even in freezing weather.

'Surgeons are macho, cold doesn't bother us', one says to her, only half-jokingly.

I am doing my obstetric training in the old Somerset Hospital in Cape Town, overlooking Granger Bay. It is the mid-1960s. I am still a medical student, and as part of my training I and the other students are expect-ed to deliver, under close supervision, as many babies as we can. But only the normal births, of course, and only African or Coloured babies – never Whites. Somerset Hospital is still there at the Waterfront, with its yellow crenellated walls and high colonial turrets, even though it was built more than a century ago, as a mid-Victorian fortress of health, and later housed casualties from the 1899-1902 Anglo-Boer War.

One night a small African woman is wheeled into the operating theatre. She is bent almost double, with a severe kyphosis of her spine.

It's a rounded deformity, a hunchback, almost certainly from past spinal tuberculosis. She also has a tiny, contracted pelvis, probably from rickets in childhood. This small woman, writhing now with labour pains, is the living embodiment of deprivation, of years of poverty and poor diet, and poor medical care, of living on the wrong side of the apartheid barrier. And now there is simply no chance, absolutely none, that she can ever have a normal birth. If she were to attempt it, the child's head would be crushed against the contracted pelvis, and after a painful and protracted labour, the baby would die – and probably so would she. About one thing there is no doubt at all: she will have to have a Caesarian Section. They wheel her swiftly into the operating theatre, the anaesthetist moves forward, and soon she is deeply asleep. But her deformed back makes it difficult for them to lay her flat on the operating table, and she lies now at an awkward, ungainly angle. The nurses drape and swab her swollen, heaving belly. Then the obstetrician, like a warrior in his green mask and gown and rubber gloves, his eyes sharp and focused, picks up his scalpel, and leans forward over her.

I look away as he makes the first incision in the skin, parting the layers of fat and muscle, and then of the uterine wall itself. But when I look back again, I catch a momentary glimpse of a small pink and purple thing, moving around within its own glistening, cellophane bag. It's like some deep-sea creature, about to rise to the surface. Then he cuts swiftly through the amniotic sac and brings forth a normal, healthy baby, wailing and yelling in the cool, disinfected air.

And soon afterwards, when they show her the baby for the first time, it is a moving, unforgettable sight – the look on her exhausted face, the smile of those toothless gums, and the tender way that she strokes and hugs the little crying, wrinkled thing. There is no chorus of angels to sing a heavenly song, no violins or harps – not in this hospital – only a circle of nurses and medical students smiling around the bed. But it's a sort of miracle, all the same.

Another hospital, elsewhere in South Africa, some years later. It is cool in the operating theatre, but the atmosphere is hot and angry. We are all arguing fiercely among ourselves, in a broken mixture of English and Afrikaans. Everyone is exhausted. It is late at night, after a long day. I am the intern, Petrus the Senior Registrar in orthopaedics, Willem the anaesthetist. There is also a theatre nurse, standing pale-faced and silent in the background. Everyone around the operating table is arguing, loudly, except for the elderly Coloured woman lying anxiously on the table between us. On her left foot, the end of her big toe is grossly infected, red and swollen. It is clear that the toenail must be surgically removed, to help clear up the infection. And yet the anaesthetist is reluctant to begin the process of anaesthesia since it will waste his precious time. Like us, he is very tired. He says it to me again:

'You don't understand. They just don't feel pain like we do, they really don't' – and Petrus nods in agreement.

They begin to swab the foot with antiseptic solution, to drape it in sterile cloths. Petrus lifts up a scalpel. That is when the argument begins again. It goes swiftly to and fro, the woman's head swivelling from one side to the other, as if at a tennis match, as it rages on above her. Eventually, I win.

'*Ag*, Willem,' says Petrus, pulling on his green mask, 'Go on, go give her the anaesthetic, then. Old Doctor Helman here doesn't believe in cruelty to animals.'

A few days later I tell my uncle what has happened. I am shaking with fury. He is a paediatrician. A kind man with white hair, a poet too.

'Write it down,' he says, Write down every detail. Otherwise, one day – when you try to tell people what happened – they won't believe you. Write it *all* down.'

'And what about that other incident?' I say, 'the one I told you about. When Petrus picked up that old Coloured guy with the bad back, and then threw him onto the examination couch, just because he was too slow climbing on to it. What about that?'

'That too,' says my uncle, 'Write it down. Every detail. Otherwise they won't believe you.'

Shortly afterwards I receive my Army papers. I have been drafted, and must report soon to an Army base in the north. I have already been through the Army medical exam – standing in line together with hundreds of other young men, while bored medics listen to my heart, feel my testicles, and get me to pee into a tall conical glass. But meanwhile the incipient guerrilla war has got hotter on the borders, especially up in South West Africa and the Caprivi Strip. As well as all this, there are continuous civil uprisings in the black townships, throughout the country. No, I think, definitely no! In fact, I am not a pacifist at all. My family served in the South African Army during the Second World War, and I would too. But to be foot-soldier of apartheid, helping to keep the Africans down in the townships? *No*, definitely not.

Only many years later do I find out that almost a third of our 1967 medical class have emigrated after their graduation, drifting out of our country, one by one – moving overseas with their families and their memories to the United States, Canada, Australia, New Zealand, Israel or England, and like me carrying with them, often guiltily, all their medical skills – and often their green masks as well.

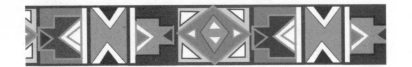

PART
2

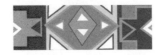

The Family
Doctor

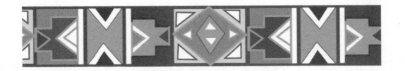

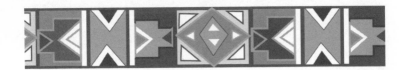

CHAPTER
6

London

After all the heat and light and space of Africa, London – with its low leaden sky and constant drizzle – is like living inside a Tupperware box, one stored deep inside a refrigerator. Everything around me is chilly, opaque, oppressive. Especially the people.

After all those years of apartheid, I am breathing the air of freedom, but it is damp and gives me chest infections. It makes me wheeze. The city is cold, and very lonely. I know hardly anyone. Furthermore, my tiny bedsit in Belsize Park, heated by its tiny gas fire, is separated by only the thinnest partition from the room next door. Night after sleepless night, sweating in my solitary bed, I can hear rhythmic grunts and long sighs, mingled with moans of ecstasy, and the banging of heads or bodies against the partition. Pillow over my head, my imagination soon develops its own form of X-ray vision. And then each time, in the post-coital calm, I hear a man's nasal, whining voice, always complaining about something, always complaining. And then a woman's voice, querulous at first, but then always apologising. And in the background, always, the sonorous rhythms of a Gregorian chant.

One day, on my way out, I notice that the door of their room has been left slightly ajar. I glance in. It is like looking into a small chapel, the air filled with powerful incense. There are two big silver candelabra on the sideboard, and on the walls framed icons, crucifixes and religious tapestries. There are big silver censers and thuribles, propped among the plaster statuettes of saints and Madonnas on the sideboard. And sitting on the bed, a young woman, staring up at me. Just before the door slams in my face, I see she is hardly wearing anything – and that she is very, very pretty. From that night on, my insomnia gets worse.

Unlike the world I knew in South Africa, the natural world doesn't seem so powerful here. The moon is tame, the stars subdued, even the sun tries hard never to shine too brightly. Dogs are on leashes, the policemen don't carry guns. In the neatly clipped trees, the birds chirp quietly among themselves in low, polite tones. There are no snakes in the suburbs, no wild animals on Hampstead Heath. With all these coiffured parks and ordered forests, Nature seems to have been firmly tamed, even human nature.

You can feel the heavy pull of the past everywhere: in the old buildings and ancient bridges, the stone castles and monuments, the old ways of behaving, and in the huge population of ghosts that pluck at your sleeve and demand attention, as they jostle and crowd every inch of this small island that they once inhabited. 'That is the curse of an old civilisation,' wrote Saul Bellow, 'It is a heavier planet. Its best minds must double their horsepower to overcome the gravitational field of tradition. Only a few will ever fly.'

A few months in London, and I have already decided to give up medicine. It seems quite as oppressive to me, as apartheid had ever been. It's clear that I am quite wrong for it, and that it's bad for me. Now finally, there's the chance to break my family script. With its Beatles and its beatniks, London in the early 1970s offers more exotic distractions than pain and penicillin. For me, the message of the city seems to be that there's a big world out there, bigger than Cape Town, but also much bigger than medicine. It's a world that doesn't only have to be about suffering and disease and how to relieve it; a novel, multi-coloured, sensual world, full of surprises, far indeed from the dour puritanism of the doctor's life.

Pregnant with some new, but still unformed identity, I grow a curly beard, then bushy sideburns, and acquire a shaggy sheepskin coat and brown bell-bottomed trousers. I begin to publish prose poems and parables in various small literary journals, and to paint illustrations for un-publishable children's books. Soon my stethoscope is firmly packed away under a high pile of poetry books. Instead of anatomical dissection or lectures on heart disease, there are plenty of poetry readings in chilly, echoing rooms above pubs, hazy with cigarette smoke. These readings, too, are mainly about the heart and about dissection, but now they are exercises in *self*-dissection by mumbling poets with wild hair and irregular teeth, who moan their couplets in these half-empty rooms, the air stale and yeasty with beer.

For a while, my poems and cartoons appear regularly in a badly printed literary journal, edited by a would-be French anarchist and poet. Jacques is a pale man dressed always in black, set off with a red Aristide Bruant scarf. He is of a type that I have never met before, certainly not at medical school: the abstract theorist, the ideas man. Like Dostoyevsky's Raskolnikov, he is young, abstract and cruel. Cold as ice. Inside his crowded head, he plots revolutions, take-overs, putsches, and the re-distribution of wealth – from 'their' pockets into his. Above the scarlet confection of his scarf, his pallid, sardonic face rests like a decapitated head – one of Madame Guillotine's more unpleasant progeny, a head amputated from its heart. Later, two friends and I edit several small surrealist literary journals with small circulations, with names like *Monsieur Dada* and *Screaming With Terror*. All this poetry makes my hair flow down to my shoulders and beyond.

My girlfriend is a student of dance and mime. I think she is quite beautiful, with her long black hair and high complexion. Our affair is intense, volatile, but there is also something detached and cinematic about it, almost literary. Inside ourselves, we are both playing on a bigger stage, and to a far bigger audience. We both come from small, remote, confined places: me from Cape Town, she from Vancouver. Now in this big, spotlit city, we feel the presence of invisible biographers, the hidden cameramen who record our every moment, the unknown journalists who one day will write about us. In the meantime there is passion. London is our *smorgasbord*. There is dance and experimental theatre, dozens of small art galleries to visit, the market at Portobello Road, the avant-garde events at the Round House theatre just down the road, the anti-apartheid rallies in Trafalgar Square, and all the expensive excitements of Carnaby Street.

I want to lead a literary, not a medical life, and now finally it's beginning to happen. For as the first year goes by, I begin to see my life summarised in bookshops, wherever I go, notated in the titles of books piled up before me: *Brave New World, The Outsider, A Separate Reality, One Hundred Years of Solitude.*

For a long while psychiatry seems the obvious option for me, especially because of my father. But I've always had this ambivalent relationship with the subject. Call it Oedipal, if you wish. In any case, I am far too fond of quoting Don Marquis's sardonic remark, that 'freuds rush in, where angels fear to tread.' But despite this scepticism, at medical school I found it easily the most attractive of all our subjects. Unlike most of our other medical tutors, at least the psychiatrists dealt with the non-material aspects of the human condition: emotions, beliefs, perceptions, memories, dreams, behaviour – not just with hormones, enzymes or the levels in the blood of this type of cell or that.

Much of my earlier attraction to psychiatry was similar to Susan Sontag's later remark about the allure of psychology: 'A large part of the popularity and persuasiveness of psychology' she wrote, 'comes from it being a sublimated spiritualism: a secular, ostensibly scientific way of affirming the primacy of "spirit" over matter'. But psychiatry is an even more secular discipline, and the absolution it offers is increasingly chemical. That's why, in those days, I find the writings of R.D. Laing so persuasive. For to me, psychiatry is not only about healing disordered minds, but also about control: about imposing a medical grid on the human condition, controlling its unruly behaviour and emotions, turning suffering into psychiatric syndromes.

Then someone suggests social anthropology. I know almost nothing about the subject, only that anthropologists are apparently people who wear pith helmets and big khaki shorts, and travel far to study remote, exotic tribes. 'Tribal experts', someone called them. But I also know that I do come from a very multi-cultural and multi-tribal society, and that I've always been fascinated by it and by its mosaic of different realities. In the early 1970s, studying the subject at London University under two famous anthropologists – Mary Douglas and Michael G. Smith – provides me with a whole new cornucopia of ideas, multiple new ways of understanding the diversity of human life. Our lectures cover every aspect of human society: their rituals, symbols, witchcraft, food taboos, the variety of religions and ways of seeing the world, the different systems of kinship and economics and political power – and especially, the different types of healer that you find world-wide, with their different forms of therapy. As the course progresses the main take-home message of anthropology, as far as I can ascertain, seems to be: 'we humans differ greatly from one another, but at the same time we are basically all the same'.

Compared with most of the doctors I know then, with their subdued clothing and muted voices, and all their talk of diseases and death, these anthropologists seem to me like brightly-coloured cockatoos, vivid and shrill with sound. Almost all of them have read interesting books, and spent time in interesting places. Over cappuccino or red Bulgarian wine, they swap tales of exotic tribes, bizarre beliefs, unusual customs.

'Well, every full moon *my* group would – '

' Yes, but that's nothing. Every week, not just every month, *my* people would sacrifice a – '

Once it was the catechism of the Latin names of muscles or the cranial nerves that fascinated me. But now it's the names of the tribes themselves – the Ndembu, the Azande, the Mai-Enga, the Khoi-Khoi, the Arapahoe, the Yaqui, and the rest – that carry with them the sounds of a chant, of an unfamiliar type of poetry. The houses or apartments my lecturers live in are lined with books. African masks, Indonesian batiks or Tibetan tankas hang on their walls. Supper is served in Zulu bowls or Indian pottery, and the bread in New Guinean basketry. There is Yemeni music on the tape recorder, or the rhythmic sounds of a Congolese Mass. They know exotic recipes. Many of the women wear heavy silver ethnic jewellery, clinking with dangling Navaho earrings, or with rows of thick Moroccan bracelets.

By comparison with these people, most doctors I know then seem more like honest craftsmen: decent, but limited. Usually no colourful tankas or Guatemalan tapestries hang on their walls. There are no Zulu bowls in their houses, no ethnic tapestries, and often very few books – except for a shelf or two of medical textbooks, a pile of telephone directories, and a few big fat paperback novels, their pages still heavily stained with suncream and sea water.

Only years later does it become apparent to me that some of these anthropologists are just as narrow and over-specialised as any medical doctor – sometimes even more so. And furthermore, they also lack that essential but unique element of the doctor: the need to *do* something, to make a difference, to try to alleviate human suffering wherever you find it. But after the traumas of apartheid and medical school, they do make me feel – for a while – that I have joined a huge global village, crowded with exotic villagers.

One day, after my graduation, this particular dream comes to a sudden end. Money is running out fast. I need to pay the rent. I don't have any money to travel, nor can I return to South Africa. And then there's a phone call from the Locum Bureau of the British Medical Association, a woman's voice, crisp and businesslike. 'Would you be interested in doing a few cruises,' she asks, 'as a ship's doctor in the Mediterranean?'

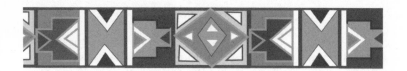

CHAPTER
7

The Rusty Ark

The brochure is shiny and vividly coloured. 'Jet away to a glistening white ship,' it urges, 'slip away through the sparkling seas of the Adriatic, the Aegean, the Tyrrhenian and the Mediterranean'. Page after page shows smiling couples – always couples – in exotic locations: the old casbah in Tunis, the slopes of Mount Etna, the port of Cagliari in Sardinia, the medieval town of Valetta. It goes on to describe the vital statistics of the ship itself: 7000 tons displacement, 3920 tons gross, overall length 372 feet, maximum speed 17 knots.

It seems a short time since I qualified and moved to England, and since I completed my studies in anthropology. This is my first 'real' medical job. Like the passengers, I've read the brochure cover to cover and am entranced by it. 'The ship will always carry an English-speaking Doctor and Nurse,' it says soothingly in its smooth, flat, laminated voice, 'and have a well-equipped surgery and hospital in case of emergency.'

But arriving aboard, having flown to Livorno from Luton, it appears that there is no hospital, no surgery, and hardly any equipment – only me, and Ngaio, the New Zealand nurse. Also on her first cruise. True, there are a few scalpels, a tin box of tweezers, clamps and catheters, some syringes and needles, a pair of forceps or two, bandages, dressings, some sterile gauze. But there are no anaesthetics, no X-ray machine, no electrocardiogram and no oxygen cylinders. On a shelf in my cabin there is a double row of bottles: antibiotics, painkillers, tranquillisers, seasickness tablets and a few other medications. Many are labelled in Greek or Italian or some other indecipherable tongue. And then there is Ngaio, as flustered and uncertain as I am. No wonder that I want to jump overboard and swim rapidly ashore. But already it is too late. The ship has cast off, and we are moving slowly, inexorably away from the quayside at Livorno. The 'Wonders of the Mediterranean' cruise has just begun.

On board there are about 450 passengers (all British), and 150 Greek crew and British tourist staff – and me; I am quite alone, except for Ngaio. With me too are my fat red copy of *Pye's Surgical Handicraft* – with its blurred black-and-white photographs of strangulated hernias and burst appendices, a second-hand copy of *Davidson's The Principle and Practice of Medicine*, and Crawford Adams's *Outline of Orthopaedics*. I read the brochure again, and scratch my head. There is no choice now. My tiny cabin on the starboard side will have to be my clinic – and also my hospital.

Many of the passengers have never before left their home towns or villages in England, let alone flown abroad for a low-budget, one-week 'cruise-jet' holiday in the Mediterranean. With every cabin fully booked, the ship is a rusty Noah's Ark of accumulated hopes, fantasies and desperate dreams. In Livorno, the first port of embarkation, the dreamers walk up the gangway, two by two, a new nightdress in the suitcase, a new hairdo, some costly perfume. There are couples trying to put new life into their stale marriages, singles hoping to find romance. For some it will work, but for others it will all end in sunburn and tears, in clumsy extra-marital gropings and beer-stained rows.

Each morning I stick a piece of hand-written paper with 'SHIP'S DOCTOR' on the cabin door, and hope that no one will knock. Then I make up my bunk, and wait for the first customers to arrive: to tell their story, to lie down upon it, and be examined.

Docking in Valetta in Malta one early morning, a middle-aged man in one of the deepest, stuffiest cabins clutches his chest and starts to pant. He is sweating and putty-faced. He says the pain is like an iron band around his chest, and in his neck and left arm. Soon, after an injection or two, he is borne quickly away by ambulance, its siren screaming. It is a heart attack. Two weeks later, in Tunis harbour, there's another man with another chest pain, vague and retrosternal. He thinks it is indigestion from too much retsina or from all the oily food. But this time, although he too is soon driven away by ambulance, it's only after a violent, gesticulating row – in French, English and Arabic – between myself and the port doctor, who disputes my diagnosis of a heart attack. (Unfortunately for the patient, I am eventually proved right).

The crew and I have an amiable but wary relationship. John, who runs the souvenir shop, comes from a mining village in the North of England. He has dark curly hair and a ready smile. Each time he meets me in the swaying corridor, he gives me the same toothy grin and knowing nudge:

'Sunk a shaft last night, Doc!'

'Oh – with whom this time?'

'Mary, that girl from Newcastle…'

He might have added: 'the one that you were also trying to get into your bunk', but he is too diplomatic for that. After all, after one of his frequent visits to those small bars on the Naples waterfront, the shadowy ones with the dim red lights, he may well have need of my medical services.

We are sailing swiftly through the Mediterranean, the sky is dark blue and misty. Livorno, Naples, Catania, Valetta, Tunis, Cagliari, Portoferraio in Elba – and then we're back to Livorno again, to pick up the next batch of tourists flown out from England. The island of Gozo glides past, wreathed in evening clouds. The weather is windy, the sea increasingly wild. The old ship heaves and creaks and strains at its rusty rivets, as it thrusts its way clumsily into the waves, like an aged lover.

Crowded onto the decks, and in the lounges and cabins, we are like patients in Somerset Maugham's story *Sanatorium*. A suffering Ship of Fools, with almost everyone (me included) trying to recover from something: a relationship, a marriage, a stressful job, a dead-end affair. Like any sanatorium, the ship floats in a timeless zone, free of the constraints of ordinary life, a rusty ark full of dreams. My work goes on.

Meanwhile, the band members are drinking themselves slowly to death – their livers are in a mess. They are all faded, wrinkled men, with smokers' coughs and high blood pressure. The pianist in the band sits on my bunk, his fingers fidgeting in his lap. They are long and angular, stained dark khaki at their ends: pianist's fingers, with the first small buds of osteo-arthritis beginning to bloom at their distal joints. His old tuxedo smells of tobacco, its elbows are worn. He coughs into a stained handkerchief. He has gastritis and heartburn again – and liver problems. His duodenal ulcer is playing up. He says that he drinks to forget, but also to remember. For, many years ago he was the pianist in the backing group of a famous male singer, so famous that everyone on board, I am sure, has danced to his music or else whistled his tunes. Now only the pianist's chest is whistling, with emphysema. The rest of him is increasingly pale, the skin clammy. On the walls of his tiny, cramped cabin, the old posters and photographs have begun to peel off in the damp air. They're all that remains, he says.

Over the weeks, I see many other cases in my cabin. A man with gall-stones, in terrible pain; some women with urinary tract infections; several other people with heartburn, from too much ouzo or retsina; a few episodes of blood pressure, either too high or too low; a possible outbreak of glandular fever among the pale cabin boys in the ship's bowels. There's seasickness galore, especially in the Straits of Messina (or so I hear from Ngaio, for I am too busy being sick myself to help anyone else). There's lots of sunburn, sometimes appearing in unexpected parts of the body. There are sexual dysfunctions of every variety (including some neither I nor my textbooks have ever heard of). There are strained wrists and twisted ankles, a broken toe and a dislocated thumb. There are a dozen or so insect bites. There's boozy weeping after boozy marital rows. There's sobbing and nightmares after a series of bag-snatchings in Catania and Naples by young men who whiz past on speedy Lambrettas. And then there's the occasional unique souvenir of Naples nightlife: the painful, discharging genitals of one of the crew members. On the last cruise, staggering along the wet, swaying decks, I take to wearing a long brown jellaba against the cold, bought in Sidi Bou Said. No wonder they nickname me 'Doctor Jellaba'.

Ships are never democracies. They are small floating autocracies, where the Captain is always king. On each of the cruises our Captain practises *droit du seigneur* on one of the latest crop of divorcees who come aboard at Livorno. He usually keeps watch from the upper deck as a line of women with peroxided hair, big earrings, and hard disappointed faces totter unsteadily up the gangway on their high-heeled shoes. And each cruise I sit at the Captain's table opposite the latest one, and watch as she gradually begins to relax and soften and then to flower, smiling, clinking glasses with the Captain, while behind her through the portholes the blue horizon drifts dreamily by. And then usually, on the last day, I watch her walk slowly down the gangway, snuffling into a tissue, as the mascara runs thickly down her cheeks like melted tar.

Early one morning, as I am returning from a visit to a sick patient in their cabin, there is a sudden loud crummp, and the usual background throb of the engines falls silent. Apparently they have over-heated, and a boiler has flooded in the engine room. It happens just as we are entering the Bay of Sorrento. A few minutes later, as the crew struggle to do temporary repairs, there is a near collision with two other ships crossing our path. Everyone is tense, some of the crew are shouting. My friend Yannis, the First Officer, explains to me that the ship was once a small French cargo vessel, bought cheaply second-hand. It has also been refitted by the new owner on the cheap, the holds converted into dozens of cramped, stuffy cabins with poor ventilation and thin metal walls. To save even more money, it has not been dry-docked nearly often enough to remove all the barnacles encrusted on its hull. These roughen its surface, says Yannis, and slow the ship down, forcing its engines to strain even harder to get to port on time – to meet the tourist company's deadlines and the fleet of tour buses that wait for us at every quayside.

'He tries always to save money,' says Yannis, 'so he causes to us always much, much trouble.'

Two weeks later, there is another explosion (in which one of the engineers burns his arm severely), and for eight hours we float help-lessly off Cape Bon in Tunisia. While the crew again fight to repair her, the British passengers play bingo and cards in the lounge, and the Greek Captain and crew marvel at their sangfroid. Meanwhile I, with my South African passport (barred then from North Africa and most other places), spend my time debating whether or not I should first throw myself or my passport overboard, if we get any closer to shore.

In Naples during one cruise, a male passenger is put ashore after a painful attack of gallstones. With officials of the tourist company, I visit him later in the Ospedale Garibaldi. It is my first experience of another type of hospital, one totally different from those I've experienced in Britain and South Africa. For here (as in many African,

Asian and Latin American hospitals), the hospital and community are not split so far apart as they are in the northern countries. In the Ospedale, the community, village and family all spill into the hospital. They cluster noisily around their relative's bed, touching, kissing, reassuring, arguing, feeding, even praying together. They surround the patient with affection and the sound of familiar voices. They help keep his or her sense of identity intact at this anxious time. The nurses' main job, as far as I can see, is only to dispense medicines, give injections, and take blood pressure and pulse rate at regular intervals. It's not that great for infection control, but how very different the atmosphere is from all those emotionally cold North European hospitals I've visited, with their patients ripped out of family and community, stripped of all signs of their personal identity, then put to bed in a long echoing ward, in a uniform of pyjamas or bed-robe. They lie alone, at an anxious time, among a crowd of other anxious strangers. The visit to the Ospedale, and subsequent visits in Brazil, Africa and elsewhere, show me that hospitals don't have to be like that, that they can be made less impersonal (even if this means, sometimes, making them more chaotic), and that the patient's family and community should always be regarded as allies in his or her treatment, not as enemies or intruders.

The ship is also my very first ever experience, after medical school, of the essential solitude of the doctor. I learn what it is like to be the only healer, as well as moral adviser, for a small, bounded community: to hold the health of that community in my hands and make crucial decisions, all on my own; to decide whom to treat and exactly how; to know what to say to ill people and how to say it; to be able to tell bad news as well as good; and to be a repository of other people's secrets, their dreams and whispered fears. It's a precious and intimate bond, and I welcome it, though it's nerve-racking at times. But when there's no one else to do it, you just have to grow into the job, break through the wall of fear. It's an essential part of becoming a doctor – to jump out of the textbook page, and then land, forcefully, in the real world.

And on each new cruise, as the crew casts off the long mooring ropes and the little rusty ship of dreams drifts slowly away from the concrete quay at Livorno, that little community is formed once again. And for another week, at least, I am their only doctor. Me – and *Pye's Surgical Handicraft*.

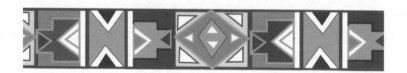

CHAPTER
8

Possession

I am back on dry land doing my rounds. Suzie is only about 11 years old, but somehow she terrifies me. I have never experienced this before, this fear of a child – and only a thin and fragile child at that, weak, ailing and bed-ridden. Certainly this terror is not something a junior doctor working for a short time in a paediatric ward should feel. And yet Suzie *is* terrifying – to others, as well as to me. It is her gruff voice, her random snarls and gruntings, her wild hair and bulbous rotating eyes, and the thick, bitter, fishy odour that always surrounds her body, no matter how often the nurses sponge her down. Ever since she first lunged at me, clawing at my eyes with her overgrown finger-nails as I leaned over her bed, I have tried to avoid her. Now she lies restlessly, heavily sedated, her bed surrounded with metal gates on either side, while a dark stain of urine spreads slowly between her legs.

There is something else that I find terrifying about her. It is that atavistic impulse that I feel rising inside me each time I hear her snorting or snarling, or see her wild, vicious clawing movements. It rises like a toxic larva from somewhere deep within myself: the instinct to stone her, smash her, to burn and destroy. It's as if she were possessed by something malevolent, invisible. It's shameful, this primitive echo within myself, but I know that I am not the only one in the ward who feels it.

And when, sometime later, after many detailed tests, the solution to Suzie's bizarre behaviour is eventually revealed, the feeling remains. Poor Suzie is not possessed by some malevolent demon. It's all due to a brain tumour, one sited in an unusual part of the brain and which shortly will be removed, hopefully completely, by a skilful neurosurgeon. Given the uncomfortable feelings that she provokes in all of us, it's fortunate for Suzie that she wasn't born in the Middle Ages, or in some parts of Africa or Asia today. Nor in Salem, Massachusetts, or in the eastern counties of England during the great 'witch craze' of the 16th and 17th centuries, when many thousands of women and girls, some probably much like Suzie, were accused of being witches, of being possessed by the Devil or his demonic servants, the succubi or incubi – and were then tortured and publicly burned alive.

Actually, our reaction to Suzie's condition is, sad to say, not that unusual. Her case reminds me that the idea of 'possession' causing disease, bodily changes or a change in behaviour seems to be universal, and always provokes the same unease in those around the victim. Anthropologists have reported this phenomenon from many different societies worldwide; historians, too. But in different places it shows itself in different ways: as possession by malevolent 'spirits' or 'demons' in one society, 'witchcraft' or 'voodoo' in another, or a particular god in a third. Back in the Middle Ages, for example, epilepsy (known then as the 'sacred disease') was often blamed on possession by evil spirits, and in desperation prayers for its relief were offered to St Valentine, St Vitus or St Sebastian. For still today, even in the Western world, many people believe the skin is porous, the body's boundaries permeable to outside forces that can cause disease, or death: whether they are demons or *jinns*, witchcraft or the Evil Eye, or even the natural environment itself. Today we're not supposed to believe in possession any more, but phrases such as 'What's got into you?', 'He drove like a man possessed', or even the word 'enthusiasm' (from the Greek, 'the God within') are distant echoes of this belief.

That's why the elderly man sitting across the desk from me – coughing, shivering and blowing his nose, seems so odd. Newly arrived in chilly England from sunny South Africa, I have never before heard that phrase that he's just used: 'Feed a cold, starve a fever'. What does he mean by it? Or by his emphatic assertion that his 'colds' and 'chills' are due mostly to Nature – particularly cold, damp, wind, ice or rain – which has somehow 'entered' or 'penetrated' his body and made him ill. You can 'catch a cold' by 'sitting in a cold draught', he says, or by 'getting caught in the rain' (especially without a hat on), 'stepping onto the cold floor after a hot bath', or even 'going outside from a hot house into the cold air'. It's not quite the same as spirit possession, but many people believe that in some mysterious and invisible way cold in the environment 'enters' your body through the skin and makes it feel cold and shivery inside. Damp in the environment enters your body as fluid, causing your nose to run, or your chest to produce phlegm. Cold causes cold, wet causes wet.

But the old man also blames his cold on his 'doing something stupid.' 'If you're not careful', he says to me, 'and you don't dress warmly enough, then the cold will get right into your body and make you ill, that's for sure. And then it'll give you a cold or even a chill'. That's the time apparently to 'feed a cold' – to make yourself so warm inside, that you prevent or 'starve a fever'.

In the long, damp, misty English winters, many of the patients in this middle-class suburb frequently get respiratory illnesses: coughs, colds, sniffles, sinusitis, flu, bronchitis, even pneumonia, especially the elderly. But almost a century after the bacteriological discoveries of Pasteur and Koch, Nature is still seen as the main culprit.

These elderly folk remind one that before 'germs' were discovered, most diseases were blamed on Nature (and before that on 'possession' by evil spirits or the Devil, or on divine punishment or just 'bad fortune'). But by the 19th century not only draughts, chills, damp, heat and rain were thought to make you ill, but also the so-called 'miasmata' – the 'bad air', foul-smelling and noxious, that was believed to be given off by stagnant ponds, human wastes, rotting vegetables or decomposing animals. In fact everything in the environment, according to the medical historian Roy Porter, that was 'filthy and putrescent', especially the poisonous vapours of the over-crowded slums, could make you ill. That was the reason, most believed, that the poor got ill more frequently than the rich.

But if Nature was largely the cause, then it was also part of the cure.

In the Victorian age and before, 'fresh air', sea, wind, water, sun and natural mineral waters were all believed to have healing properties. Many hospitals had their own glass-walled 'solarium', where patients could be exposed for hours on end to the healing rays of the sun. Even today the *kur* in Germany and *la thermalisme* in France are popular for their health-giving waters and steam, just as such spas once were throughout Great Britain and the USA. Pale tubercular people – like those in Thomas Mann's novel *The Magic Mountain* – were often sent off to recover in 'sanatoria', far from the noxious air of the big, polluted, overcrowded cities. There they would spend months, or even years, in small sealed-off communities in the cool pellucid air of the Alps or in the dry desert air of Arizona. In this setting Nature could work its wonders in alliance with human nature and with the human body. But one of the most powerful forces of Nature was always *time* – the true healer, the one with which the wise doctor always works in alliance. Time would kill some, but it would also heal many others.

Then in the late 19th century, 'possession' made a comeback, though in an unexpected form. For Louis Pasteur's experiments in the 1880s showed that many diseases aren't due to Nature at all (or to evil spirits or demons or bad-smelling air), but to micro-organisms – tiny, invisible, dangerous things that enter the body and make you ill. And shortly after him, Koch discovered the tuberculosis bacillus in 1882 and the cholera bacillus in 1883. Despite this history of medical discoveries, scientific knowledge seems to seep very slowly into people's minds, especially here in Europe. In this particular leafy suburb in London, I have seen how scientific germ theory is only now percolating into parts of the popular consciousness. And there's a clear, generational difference, for it's the younger people who embrace it most enthusiastically. These days they almost always blame those same 'colds' and 'chills' on invisible creatures they call 'germs'.

For most of them, though, 'germs' is just a word – really just a hypothesis, a theory of causality – and not quite the same tiny entities as those familiar to Koch, Pasteur and the bacteriologists of today; or the ones I peered at under the microscope in my medical school days back in Cape Town. Hardly any of my patients have ever actually seen a 'germ', whether in a book or under the microscope. They're not even sure what they look like, nor what they do, nor how they actually cause you to be ill. They often confuse 'germs', 'bugs' and 'viruses', using the words interchangeably, and thus demand antibiotics (inappropriately) for all three of them. They describe these 'germs' to me as invisible, malevolent entities that somehow 'enter' your body by its orifices, and then make you ill. They make you cough and sneeze, and give you a fever or a rash or diarrhoea, or something even worse. And each 'germ' seems to have its own recognisable and unpleasant 'personality' of symptoms by which it reveals itself once it has entered you ('I've got that one, Doctor, you know – the one that gives you the dry cough, the watery eyes, the runny nose, and the shivering'). Often it's one that is currently 'going around' the area, the office or the school.

'Yes, yes,' I say, nodding, 'I know the one. You're right, it *is* going round the area. This week I've seen lots of cases of it already. '

They look relieved. They are 'normal' after all. Most importantly, it's not really their fault. It's all those damned bugs and malevolent viruses out there, not them. Blaming a 'germ' makes them more a victim of external forces, of 'possession' by some external entity, rather than someone responsible for their own illness. And it matches neatly all the many other ways that they increasingly tend to blame all their misfortunes on others: their parents, their spouses, their employers, the state.

What fascinates me is that these British folk ideas of 'germs' are not so dissimilar to more traditional ideas of 'spirit' possession, described by anthropologists from many parts of the developing world. Ioan M. Lewis, for example, has described how in many rural African societies, disease is still blamed on 'disease-bearing spirits', invisible, malevolent entities that somehow enter your body, 'possess' you and then make you ill. He writes that among people like the Luo of Kenya, disease is often blamed on amoral, malicious spirits who 'possess' their victims in a capricious and unpredictable way, while among followers of the *bori* cult of the Hausa people in Nigeria, each spirit – like each 'germ' in London – is associated with a particular cluster of symptoms, such as pain, fever, cough or bleeding. There too, 'spirits' are hypotheses, theories of causality, invisible entities believed to cause suffering or illness, and which wait in ambush at the periphery of every human life.

Back in suburban London, 'possession' ideas have certainly not disappeared, despite all the wonders of modernity and the many discoveries of medical science. And they exist still not only in folk theories of 'germ' infection, or in the origins of 'colds' and 'chills'. They also exist in liquid form. I think of the word 'spirits' – commonly used in Britain to describe strong drinks such as whisky, brandy or vodka.

'I know that it's not him talking that way, Doctor', says the battered wife of the alcoholic to me one day, her hand held tightly over her bruised cheek, 'I know that it's not. It's the spirits talking, not him. It's all those spirits that he drinks, saying those horrible, hurtful things to me. And then hitting me like that. It's just them, Doctor, it's not him. Believe me, I know him, and I love him, and it's not his fault. It's the spirits inside him. And besides, he really *needs* me… '

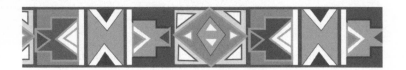

CHAPTER
9

Suburban Tales

It's just an ordinary English suburb, an area of semi-detached houses, many pseudo-Tudor in style, with dark parallel beams in their white walls and latticed windows. Each has its own tiny front garden, surrounded by low trimmed hedges and modest topiary. On every side of the Medical Centre where I am working, the roads and avenues of the suburb are lined with these neat rectangles of lawn, adorned with ivy, honeysuckle and climbing roses, and with beds of pansies, marigolds, hollyhocks and gladioli. On summer weekends, husbands in T-shirts and rolled-up sleeves can be seen sweating and puffing, as they paint or hammer, or push roaring lawnmowers across their little postage stamps of lawn. Some of the front gardens are designed as a mini-Versailles, with small stone statues, tiny fishponds, a miniature fountain or two, and ornamental bowers of wire or wood.

Meanwhile, in the houses and gardens, wives and children mill around. Music throbs from the rooms of teenagers, their walls plastered with brightly coloured posters. Rows of family cars and station wagons are parked in driveways or line the sides of the road. On most afternoons, a few children can be seen cycling along the broad streets lined with different types of tree: horse chestnut, sycamore, prunus and ash. Very few single people live in the area, for it is one favoured mainly by couples. It's an area of semi-detached houses, occupied by people living semi-detached lives – joined together at the heart, like Siamese twins.

Within this area there's a new and rising population of young *nouveaux riches*, richly dressed and expensively coiffured, which spends much energy and time on competition: who has the newest car, the biggest breasts, the largest kitchen, the prettiest children. Many of them seem obsessed with the surfaces of things. They talk at length, and in minute detail, about scratches on their cars, stains on their carpets, a weed in the lawn. Sitting anxiously on a chair in my consulting room, they have long conversations with me about minor rashes on their faces, microscopic pimples, the faintest of blemishes beyond the bikini line, the very slightest asymmetry between one earlobe and the other ('Can't you see, Doctor? Can't you see how *different* they are?'). Their houses, too, are temples of Order: ivory white walls, light cream carpets, all the surfaces shiny as mirrors, and that ubiquitous tang of deodorants, air-fresheners and furniture polish.

Order, cleanliness, symmetry: everything in its place. But why are so many people in the suburb so unhappy? Why do they take so many tranquillisers or anti-depressants? Why do they smoke so heavily or drink too much?

And yet behind these ordered gardens and regulated rose bushes, behind the lace curtains, lies a rich and secret life. Even as a family doctor it takes a long time to discover it – in my case, several years – but it's actually a world of vivid characters and stifled dreams, of hidden paranoia and frustration and odd obsessions, of wild ambitions that can never be fulfilled and passionate affairs doomed to disaster, of hundreds of secret selves hidden carefully behind hundreds of bourgeois masks. Behind the lace curtain petticoats and neatly trimmed hedges there are scores of people living shadow lives as suburban *femmes fatales*, local Svengalis, amateur actors or actresses, unusual hobbyists, minor sports heroes, neighbourhood potentates or curious eccentrics. As their family doctor, it's reassuring to find out eventually that it's a world just like any other – only more so.

'Doctor, there's little silver fish in my urine again.'

'*What*? What did you say about your urine?'

'There's little silver fish, Doctor, in the toilet, every time I take a pee. Swimming around in there. Tiny little things – about this long.'

The gruff smoker's voice on the telephone trails away. I imagine Mrs N holding her gnarled arthritic thumb and index finger an inch or so apart, just in front of the phone. For a moment I recall all those lectures on tropical medicine that I attended at medical school in Cape Town. All those diagrams of exotic parasites projected onto the screen of the crowded lecture theatre: the life cycle of *Plasmodium vivax*, the curious cytoplasm of *Entamoeba histolytica*, the wiggly flagellae of *Giardia intestinalis* or the liver fluke – and all those lectures on other tropical parasites – yaws and yellow fever, leprosy and taeniasis, amoebiasis and ankylostomiasis. Could she have picked up one of them? Or the larvae of bilharzia, maybe? Has she ever been to the tropics? To any part of Africa? I page quickly through the thick wad of her medical notes. No, impossible. It looks like she has never left England, probably never even left the suburb in which she was born. What can it be?

She is still waiting for me at the other end of the line, wheezing heavily into the receiver.

'I know that you don't believe me, Doctor,' she says, ' I know you think that I'm making it all up, that I'm crazy and all that, but I passed some more this morning. Into a chamber pot. And this time I've kept them for you to see!'

I can hardly wait. After the morning clinic, my car leaps through the crowded streets to her little house like an eager stallion, as keen to get there as I am. Already I am framing my letter to *The Lancet*. A new disease! A rare, parasitic disease, discovered here in suburbia. My name attached to it, of course. Or should my report be sent instead to the *New England Journal of Medicine*?

I bang loudly on her door, its paint chipped and peeling. Somewhere in the bowels of the house, I can hear Mrs N's slow, painful shuffle coming down the stairs, towards the door. She opens it, still in her dressing gown. Her hair is a wild explosion of yellow and white. And she's forgotten to put her teeth in this morning. She says nothing. Her face is empty. She leads me slowly up the stairs, the carpets dusty and torn. On the first landing is a small wooden table and, resting on it, a large porcelain chamber pot, covered with a plate. She moves towards it. Her smile is wide, toothless with triumph.

'Here it is, Doctor,' she says, 'ready for you to see. Go on, have a look at them.'

She lifts up the plate. I look eagerly in. The pot is empty – except, of course, for urine. No fish.

Mrs N shakes her head in wonder. Her naked gums make a tut-tut-tut sound.

'Damn!' she says, 'Those cunning little things. Well, what do you know? What do you know? They've done it again! Gone and slipped out from under the plate while I was going downstairs to open the door for you. Well what do you know? Clever little swine aren't they, eh? *Damn!*'

Mr A rolls his eyes. He peers at me sideways, lids half-closed, and then swiftly scans the consulting room above and behind me, his reddened eyes rotating in his balding head like two terrified goldfish inside a bowl. I take out a pen and a piece of paper, and together we add them all up, one by one. All the people whom he says are 'watching' him, keeping him under surveillance, following him, bugging his decrepit old house in the leafy cul de sac, listening to his every whisper.

Firstly, there are those disguised as 'neighbours': I calculate seven people in all. Then there are the two so-called 'policemen', in their fake uniforms who 'patrol' outside his house at the same time every morning. Then there's that bogus 'milkman', pretending to deliver his 'milk' (but really, his miniature bugging devices) to the 'neighbour' next door. There's those two men, clumsily disguised as 'postmen'; several 'mothers' and their supposed 'children'; two imitation 'street sweepers'; a man on a bicycle who always wears a blue pullover ('Yes, he wears the same pullover every day; it's a type of signal to the others'); and several hefty men, pretending to repair the road even though, week after week, the road never seems to become repaired. I add them all up. Excluding the 'children', that makes twenty-three.

'Twenty-three people, Mr A,' I say, 'Twenty-three! That's an awful lot of people. It must cost someone a fortune to hire them all, don't you think? Who could possibly afford all that expense, on a daily basis? You tell me.'

But it's not working. Science, rationality, argument, numbers – all useless. Mr A shrugs. He leans forward, glances uneasily around him, then lowers his voice to a whisper:

'It's the American Embassy,' he says, 'They're behind it.'

'But *why*?' I cry out, 'Why would the American Embassy possibly spend all that money, and send all those people, just to keep you under observation. Why you? Are you that important?'

Mr A looks at me with pity. He shakes his head. He explains slowly, carefully, as if to a child.

'You know that I told you some years ago that I was divorced, Doctor, and that my wife lives overseas now. Well, you know, I heard recently that she has re-married.'

'So?'

'So – she married an American. That's the answer! That's my point. Now do you see what I mean?'

I fall back in my chair, and reach for my prescription pad. For him or for me? That is the question.

Mr A gets up and begins his slow shuffle out of the room. At the doorway, he suddenly turns and then looks back at me, suspiciously. His eyes are rotating wildly again.

'Come to think of it, Doctor,' he says frowning, 'Come to think of it – why are you asking me all these questions today? Why have *you* become so interested in knowing so much about *me*?'

As the door slams behind him, I can sense the words forming in his mind – and the deep sense of satisfaction that goes with them. That one word is as clear to me as if it was printed upon his forehead, and was now blinking there in neon. Only one word:

Twenty-four!

'Good evening, Doctor. Bertram H here. Sorry to disturb you at suppertime, but I've just been to the toilet, and …'

Even today, I still feel nauseous at the very mention of his name, at the memory of that sing-song voice on the telephone, especially during mealtimes. The food on the plate before me suddenly chills, the gravy turning thick and rancid as if green fungi were growing swiftly all over it. Mr H is in his late seventies and lives alone. He is like some gentleman-scientist of the 19th century, but the only natural history that he is interested in is his own, most especially the functioning of his bowels. He phones me regularly with detailed updates: the latest shapes, sizes, textures, smells, colours, bubbles, even the condition of the water itself. He is precise, pedantic, empirical. He has all the zeal of a natural scientist, combined with that of a diviner trying to decode the messages hidden within the tarot of his own intestines

Everyone who encounters Mr H seems to dislike him, especially the receptionists who take his frequent phone calls. They talk of him with shudders and distaste. But I've gradually come to see him quite differently. For to me he is not only a scientist *manqué* or a diviner, but also a type of performance artist or even the Jackson Pollock of bodily functions. His bowel movements are his artwork, his creativity, the daily fruit of his inner self. Going to the toilet is the highlight of his day, the greatest source of novelty in a sad and solitary life, a life in which nothing ever changes. For him weeks go by in an interminable silence, broken only by the distant crackle of the radio, without a visit or a conversation, a touch or a telephone call. His small house is like a waxworks museum, frozen in time. It is dusty, unchangeable, embalmed ever since his wife died there many years ago. It is filled with ancient furniture and elderly magazines. There's an old yellowed fridge with thick enamelled walls and a big silver handle, coughing and pulsing in the kitchen, and an elderly bakelite 'wireless' standing in one corner of the crowded lounge. Standing in the centre of this ageing tableau, I can hear his voice, frail but insistent:

'Doctor, I'm still in the toilet. Please come in here. The door's unlocked. I just want to show you something. Something *very* interesting …'

It's my very first time inside a convent, and so I'm very ill at ease. (After all, what do *I* know about convents?) They've called me in to see a Sister Bernadette, who's apparently got the flu. I walk through the arched gateway and knock nervously on the thick, bolted, double-door with its heavy oak beams. I'm still in my early days in London, and doing a short locum in the area, covering for an elderly doctor who's away on sick leave. As usual I am wearing my blue Royal Air Force-surplus coat, my bell-bottomed trousers and wide striped tie, and my beard is still curly and untrimmed.

In the entrance hall to the convent, smelling of floor polish and festooned with big vases of flowers, crucifixes and holy pictures, Sister Mary is waiting for me. I recognise her voice: she is the one who had phoned me. She says that Sister Bernadette is feeling quite poorly today. She says that she will take me up to her room. As she is greeting me, the Mother Superior walks into the entrance hall, a tiny Mother Teresa look-alike, with a round face and thick rimless glasses. She looks me up and down.

'Will you be fixing it here,' she asks slowly, ' or will you be wanting to carry it away with you?'

Take Sister Bernadette away? Carry her away? On my shoulders? How much does she weigh? Is this what doctors in England usually do? And why does she call her an 'it'? Don't say that she's… that I've come too late … that she's just – *Oh No!*

Suddenly, Sister Mary intervenes.

'He's the doctor, Mother,' she says gently, ' the *doctor*. Not the television repair man.'

Old Mr J, with sunken cheeks and blue sparkling eyes, leans towards me across the desk and whispers a toothless secret into my ear. He smells of old soap and tobacco and musty clothing.

Together with other elderly folks, he tells me, he regularly attends a Day Centre a few miles away. It's a large building, with good facilities, where for one or two days a week they are well cared for and fed, or entertained, while some do keep-fit or play bingo or cards, or even take dance classes. Some, but not all of them, have mental health problems. A few even have severe depression or psychosis: sad, shadowy people, often ignored by their families or even by the carers who are paid to look after them. They are often difficult or cantankerous or confused. Some are prone to violent, toothless rages. Others are increasingly unsteady on their feet, or even incontinent. Many have been broken by terrible life experiences. But most of those who attend the Day Centre are just very old and very forgetful.

I've never visited there, but I've always thought of it as a rather depressing place, an institution – terminal, soulless, grey, a modern Dickensian dumping ground for the frail and the unwanted. But old

Mr J, his eyes twinkling, gums chuckling, bald head shaking with mirth, tells me I am wrong. Completely wrong! He chuckles colour and movement back into the black-and-white picture that I have created of the place. He tells me that there's a vibrant life in the Centre, one that I know absolutely nothing about, a shadow world hidden from view: not only one of romances, friendships, intricate feuds and slow-motion flirtations, but also a secret economy. For in the halls and toilets of the Day Centre, a complex network of exchanges takes place: a roaring trade in sedatives, anti-depressants, sleeping tablets and other medicines. For a day or two a week, in this hidden little world, many of the old people have recreated in miniature their old identities, stolen from them by years of institutionalisation. Here, merchants once more become merchants, traders become traders again, and entrepreneurs can still play the market, searching for the Perfect Deal. Some act as wholesalers, others as retailers or even as travelling salesmen – staggering furtively on their Zimmer frames across the hall from group to group, their pockets filled with sleeping tablets.

Without the knowledge of nurses or carers, the Day Centre apparently functions as an unofficial bourse, with its own specific rates of exchange ('I'll give you two Prozac's for one Seroxat. *That's* the deal.'). Mr J assures me, his face serious now, that in almost every case the drugs are not swapped in order to be swallowed, but only for the sake of the exchange itself. They are traded and then re-traded, like stocks and shares in some phantom pharmaceutical company, or an informal version of Petticoat Lane Market.

Of course, I alert the Day Centre to what is going on. But even as I put down the telephone, I know that it will make no difference. For even if they are strictly forbidden, the surreptitious exchanges will continue to take place. As long as the elderly merchants and the toothless entrepreneurs have got one breath left in their frail, trembling bodies – and as long as they are able to remember exactly how many Prozac are worth how many Seroxat, they will continue to trade them, or else switch to trading cigarettes or tubes of toothpaste.

So I was wrong. Their lives are not over yet. Hidden behind the trembling masks of senility, life goes on: busy, vibrant, absorbing, chockfull of energy and shrewd calculation. In fact, a life much like our own.

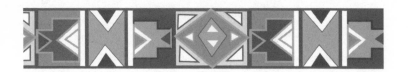

CHAPTER
10

Déformation
professionelle

I think of Mr R. Who could ever forget him? He of the elongated black moustache, its waxed ends curled and twirled elaborately into the air like Arabic calligraphy. An unusual-looking man in his late seventies or early eighties, he is bald and bullet-headed, short, powerfully built. He usually wears a fat multicoloured tie, a homburg hat, and an old-fashioned grey suit with wide lapels. His accent is from somewhere in the north of England. Today is the first time that I ever met him, and with his curious clothes Mr R reminds me of some recently-retired *apparatchik* from Central Europe or maybe of someone just escaped from the set of a 1930s gangster movie. Either way, it's not only his looks that are unusual, but also his way of talking. Or rather of barking. For each time he replies to my questions about his symptoms, he emits a loud, forceful sound – his voice somewhere between a thunderous yell and a very loud, angry bark, one that grows louder every moment.

'Doctor, I think it began about four weeks ago, (BARK! BARK!) Coughing and coughing and coughing. Always wheezing every night, for hours on end. (BARK!) I can't sleep a wink because of it. No sleep at all'. (BARK! BARK! BARK!).

'So, tell me again, Mr R, how many cigarettes did you say you've been smoking recently? Per day?'

'How many? Not many, Doctor, as I've just said to you. Only thirty or forty. Who knows? I roll my own. It's not the smoking. It doesn't harm me.

(BARK!) My chest is strong. (BARK!) Always has been. Very strong. (BARK! BARK! BARK!).'

But my stethoscope tells a different story, one narrated in the tell-tale expiratory wheezes and whistles of chronic bronchitis. Not surprisingly, he has a deep, cavernous cough, and the sounds of his breathing are remote and stifled. And it's impossible not to spot, in the big-barrelled shape of his chest, the unmistakable sign of emphysema. For a moment I wonder whether he is what doctors call a 'pink puffer' or a 'blue bloater'. And then there's the revealing state of his fingertips, for the ends of these ten thick hairy sausages, covered with rings, are all stained a yellowish brown.

Mr R makes me angry. His type always does. He has severe emphysema and recurrent bronchitis, so why won't he just stop smoking? Why won't he just look after himself? Why is he so damned self-destructive? It makes me so angry that I begin to roar my displeasure at him, to bark back at him. My voice is harsh and accusing. I can feel myself rising from my chair, my face livid with rage, still roaring. Why won't he just *stop* smoking?

Suddenly, I stop. For I become aware of something new in the room. For Mr R is now staring fixedly at me, and his bark has become even louder. Furthermore, he seems to be emanating some powerful force-field. It's invisible, of course, but I can still feel it flowing across the desk towards me, pushing me back, forcing me back into my chair. Even trying to remember my earlier karate training and doing slow deep abdominal breathing, I have difficulty in forcing it back. For a while I hold it at bay at the edge of my desk. I strain and push. He pushes back. The struggle is invisible, but exhausting. I can feel myself beginning to fade. Several times, asking him about this symptom or that, I notice how my voice itself seems to be fading away. With surprise I watch as it drops off its perch, and falls helplessly through the air like a wounded bird, wings beating fainter with every second.

And then I become aware of a second, very unusual sensation in the small of my back. It's a pain, or rather three different pains, each one arranged vertically, and in parallel. I realise what is happening. It's as if some big meaty hand has been pushing me backwards, pressing my body so firmly against the upright part of my chair that its three wooden struts have been digging deeply into my back.

Eventually Mr R leaves the room, clutching his prescription for antibiotics and a bronchodilator spray. I fall back exhausted into my chair. My chest is aching. And my back pain is still there – in triplicate.

Who is Mr R? What is he? I search frantically through his medical file, a bulging tan folder filled with scrawled cards and typed letters, many of them written to his previous doctors. Eventually I come across one letter, many years old, which gives me the answer. As I read the faded paper, I realise that Mr R has spent most of his working life inside an unusual world, one far removed from most people's everyday lives. For a moment, I recall that certain sadness that seemed to settle on his flushed wheezing face, between each defiant bark. For compared to his glorious past he is nothing now, only a sick old man in the suburbs with a very bad chest, and arthritis in every joint. But once, a very long time ago, he was something else, something much more. In fact, his particular story permeates much of our literature and myth, from the Bible onwards: the stories of Daniel and Samson, of Gilgamesh and Captain Ahab, of St George and his dragon. Even of the Iberian toreadors of today. It's the archetypal story of the Hero and of his transcendent triumph over the wild, unruly forces of Nature, of Man over Beast.

Ever since childhood I have been drawn to Mr R's world, that small circular, archetypal landscape. I have sought it out in Cape Town, and Johannesburg, and even in London. For it's really one of the last remaining refuges of our mythic imagination, a world of archetypes, the one first nurtured by our ancestors around their ancient campfires. It is a place of heroism, bathos, humour and fear, incandescent with glittering lights and thunderous applause, where the laws of space and time are for a while wholly suspended. It is a place where animals do impossible things, where men and women fly gracefully through the air like birds, and gravity is defied.

I read again the beginning of the letter, written over a decade ago by a chest specialist to his then family doctor.

'Dear Dr Williams – ' it reads – 'Thank you for referring this 65-year old retired lion tamer, who is a very heavy smoker… '

I guess you just have to get used to it, in family practice: the way that some people bring not only their illnesses to you, but also their *déformation professionnelle* – the way that their professions have shaped, and deeply influenced them, over very many years. And it's not only retired lion-tamers, either. There's the ex-army officer, for example, barking out commands at me from across the desk ('I need a new prescription, Doctor, and I'm afraid I need it *now!*'). The policeman, eyeing me suspiciously as I ask about his symptoms, then questioning me closely on my comments ('Now hold on a moment, Doctor, hold on a moment, what *exactly* do you mean by saying that it's all due to my liver?'). The school teacher, lecturing me about the exact, and precise, nature of his bowel symptoms ('Now do you understand what I've been trying to tell you, Doctor? *Now* do you understand?"). The lawyer, cross-questioning me about the results of his blood tests ('Now what precisely do you mean by that, Doctor? Could you be more specific, please, and define it rather more clearly, if you please?'). The business man bargaining ('Look, Doc, I'll make a deal with you. I'll cut out salt and fatty foods and promise to go to the gym regularly, if you'll just reduce my blood pressure tablets. How about that?').

Patients bring their *déformation professionnelle* with them to the doctor, and you have to work within it. You have to sense, and understand, the system of metaphors and meanings and practices that dominate their lives, and then frame your medical advice in those terms, in a way that makes sense to them.

I remember once doing a locum in a general practice in an affluent area of central London. I found it to be full of big confident men in dark three-piece suits, with loud confident voices: stockbrokers, top executives, big businessmen, senior managers, CEOs of this multinational or of that. But I also found them almost impossible to deal with because their lifestyles were so self-destructive. They drank too much, smoked too much, ate too much rich food, relaxed too little, went on holiday far too seldom. They were driven, obsessed with deadlines, rushing, tense. Telling them all of this and how it might damage their health simply didn't work. They just stared at me, shrugged, and then glanced down impatiently at the big, expensive Rolex watches strapped to their wrists.

But phrase it in other terms, and their ears would prick up.

'Why don't you see your health, and your body as your capital,' I said. 'And see stopping smoking as an investment. Yes, as a long-term investment. One that in a few years time will earn you a high rate of interest. Just think of all those dividends! It's an investment that's bound to pay off! Invest in your body now – and think of all those profits that you'll earn in years to come!'

Now they were listening, closely. Slowly they would nod. *The man's talking sense*! At last! Thanking me they would lift up their big briefcases, glance quickly again at their Rolexes, and then leave. Surprisingly often it worked, sometimes not. But the principle was correct. To be a good doctor, you have to be a compassionate chameleon, a shape-shifter, a shaman. Even if your adaptation to your patients' world happens at an unconscious level, always work within their system of ideas, not against it. Even if, as with Mr R, you find yourself rising to your feet and roaring fiercely at them.

But then, on the other hand, what lion-tamer ever took advice from his lion?

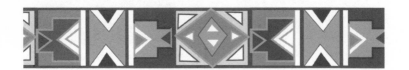

CHAPTER
11

House Calls

Tightly gripping my leather medical bag, I am walking along the chilly, echoing corridors of a big council estate. The bag is filled with an enticing collection of syringes, needles, drugs and blank prescription pads. It's a dangerous load to be carrying. These days it's no longer safe even to put a 'DOCTOR' sticker on your car windscreen in this type of poor, decaying neighbourhood. It's asking for trouble: an open invitation to the drug addicts to break into it, please, and then take just what you like. Rather get a parking ticket than face that.

I park my car next to the vandalised phone box, the one with the syringe lying on its floor and the naked wires hanging down. Inside the building, which rises ten storeys high, there is the faintest smell of urine, the throb of reggae and heavy metal from behind the double-bolted doors. The lift is out of order today. Along the ceilings the light bulbs are all in tiny metal cages, several of them broken.

Many of the draughty corridors and stairwells are decorated with big, rounded graffiti, sprayed in a bulbous calligraphy. The letters are curved and vividly coloured, and often followed by enormous exclamation marks. Something loud and emphatic is being said here, but what? I feel like an archaeologist wandering into some newly discovered tomb, its damp walls filled with inscriptions in unknown hieroglyphs.

As I climb panting up the stairs, each landing is just like the one below, with the same identical shiny purple bricks and yellowing tiles. On one landing, I step over two bags of half-eaten potato chips and a small pile of fish bones. I have been in this building many times before, visiting patients in their small flats, behind their carefully locked doors. They are small modest apartments, with family photos and mementos crowded onto the sideboards, rows of potted plants on the window sills, and the smells of cooking from the tiny kitchens. One flat, I remember, is completely bare but for a mattress on the floor and a television set booming at the centre of a large empty room.

Except for his dog, Charlie, Mr L lives alone. I think he always has done. It's the flat with the dusty windows, right on the top floor of the building, the one just next to the out-of-order lift. The back windows overlook the roofs of a nearby factory and a small empty plot, overgrown with long grass, nettles and wild flowers. Inside the flat, the central heating is always on, whatever the weather. The place is airless, stuffy, hot. And it smells. There are a few pieces of chipped furniture, a sagging bed and an old TV set that's always turned onto full volume. On the bare floor and the few tattered carpets lie high piles of yellowed newspapers, some many years old. In the kitchen, the cracked and yellowed kitchen sink is usually filled with a pile of unwashed plates, many crusted with the archaeological remains of ancient meals.

These occasional visits by me or one of my colleagues are apparently the highlight of Mr L's life. He is always very welcoming. With great courtesy and clumsy bows he always offers me sweet lukewarm tea in a chipped mug. Sometimes its thick syrupy sweetness makes me feel sick.

As always, Mr L is unshaven. And his smile when he greets me is like a broken picket fence, its slats stained and irregular. He usually wears an old dressing gown, almost as old as he is, as he shuffles and wheezes slowly around his little flat on swollen feet and flattened slippers. Under the gown he wears a string vest, but never any shirt.

Today I notice something different.

'What are those things on the floor, Johnny?' I ask, 'Over there. And what is that strong smell in the flat today?'

He looks around, and scratches his bald head. He looks puzzled.

'Oh sorry, Doctor,' he says.

He leans down and picks up, one by one, the long row of dog turds lying along the torn carpet, and then drops them into a stained red plastic bucket in the corner.

'Sorry, Doctor, it must be Charlie,' he says, and then: '*God*, it's hot in here!'

And wipes his face with his hands, and then both his eyes, and finally, slowly, the lips of his half-opened mouth.

'Sorry, Doctor,' he says again. 'Now have your tea. Here, let me give you the cup. I've just made it for you. Just before you came in.'

The housekeeper in a white blouse and long grey skirt opens the door and looks at me suspiciously, up and down. I am wearing my usual garb, the uniform of the late Sixties: the long blue RAF coat, bought from an army and air force surplus store in Camden Town, my wide multicoloured tie and brown bell-bottomed trousers, my hair and beard wild and free. I am carrying my instruments and prescriptions in my father's old leather bag. I am newly arrived in London. It's one of my very first locums in this city. I am a stranger in a strange land.

'I am the doctor, ' I announce, but even to me my voice sounds unconvincing, especially with that guttural colonial accent, 'The locum. I'm covering for Dr Craig, who is off ill today.'

Reluctantly she stands aside to let me enter. 'Lady Margaret is up in her bedroom', she says.

I walk up the long curved stairway with the gilded banisters. It is lined with family portraits, one dark oily face after another, the men in periwigs and uniforms, the women with elaborate hair-dos, each with her big brown eyes and her pale, mournful face. The faces light up the dark background, like pale candles against the gloom of death. The portraits have given the sitters a partial afterlife – something denied to most of their fellow-citizens at the time. All they had was their reflection, glimpsed for a moment in a window or in the calm surface of a village pond.

Walking up that ornate staircase is like a journey through time as well as through space. As I climb the stairs, the portraits are becoming more recent, even up to the present century. It's a walk right through

English history as well as through the history of a particular person – the one waiting for me at the top of the stairs, at the very apex of this pageant of dead faces, in her perfumed bedroom with her ankle propped up on a delicate lace cushion. It's the first time I've ever met anyone with a title.

Lady Margaret lies back on her bed, framed by a circle of large silk cushions, like an exhibit in some great museum of colonial history. She is thin and very elderly and is wearing a mask, moulded from face-powder and paint. It is white and rouged, its planes hard and angular, but without expression. The mask seems to be ageless, its eyeholes empty of clues. Standing awkwardly at the bedside I notice the hint of expensive perfume, the liver spots on her arms, the wrinkled neck, the big rings on her trembling fingers. She seems to be a woman from another age, another continent – as out of place in this modern, bustling 20th century city of London as I am. She looks me up and down. She looks baffled. She seems to be as wary of me, as I am of her. On her head she wears that pastiche of the old Raj, a silken turban. Languid among the high gilt-framed mirrors and Oriental wall-hangings, like some relic from a previous age, she resembles a wounded maharani – receiving supplicants at her private durbar.

And I am one of them, a minor servant intruding on her boudoir. She waves her hand vaguely in the direction of her foot.

'Twisted it this morning,' she says, 'Fell down the stairs. Turned it under me. Hurts like bloody hell. '

I touch it and probe it. I tut-tut-tut. I examine its bruised and swollen contours. I gently move it to and fro. For an instant, something spreads across the mask, breaking it for a second into a filigree of tiny wrinkles. 'Hurts like bloody hell,' she says again, her voice thin now and wavering.

Another woman enters the room, escorted by the housekeeper, also Lady Someone-or-Other. There is a flurry of sympathetic pecks and kisses. Another turban, another scented mask, another thin clipped accent, the words clinking and tinkling together like a glass of tiny ice-cubes. I have never heard such accents before, except on the Overseas Service of the BBC, which we tuned into in South Africa, with its faint whisper of distant voices, confident and controlled, the accents of Empire. The women chat among themselves, ignoring me. The housekeeper brings in a silver tray with a china teapot and two cups on it. I have become invisible, transparent. No one looks at me, for I am not there. No one listens as I speak on the phone to the hospital, arranging for an ambulance and for an orthopaedic specialist. No one hears me, for there is nothing at all to hear.

I pick up my bag, and walk slowly down the stairs. No one says goodbye, because no one noticed that I was ever there in the first place. On the way down, even my footsteps disappear into silence, absorbed by the thick pile of the carpeting. The portraits pass, one after another, also staring right through me. Downstairs, as I leave, the housekeeper closes the door firmly behind me. To my surprise, I find myself back in London, among the noisy black cabs and the big red buses. For a while I had thought I was somehow back in South Africa: in Johannesburg, say, among the affluent high-walled northern suburbs with their huge lawns and sprinklers and swimming pools, their rows of scented frangipani and the abundant bougainvilleas. Johannesburg of the apartheid years, where each suburban property was like a small plantation. Pausing on the front steps, I ponder on the curious resonance of our encounter, and why such an ordinary house call to a frail old lady with a damaged foot has made me so uneasy. For the world has just been turned upside down, and now – in an inversion of the apartheid world back home – I have become the Zulu garden boy, or the Basotho houseboy, as invisible and transparent and irrelevant to the rich suburban housewives as the warm scented African air that surrounds them on all sides. It's a strange and uncomfortable feeling, but one that is also curiously familiar. That world of servants. Of power and masks. And of the inner damage they can cause.

Driving away, I think of the lines of Anais Nin, in her book *Winter of Artifice*. I wonder if Lady Margaret – or the Johannesburg housewives in their similar masks of makeup – have ever read them, and the subtle warning that they contain. 'It was difficult for her to believe, as others did,' wrote Nin, 'that the mask tainted the blood, that the colours of the mask could run into the colours of nature and poison it. She could not believe that…the mask and the flesh could melt into one another and bring on infection.'

I am quite alone in the darkened room with the old woman, holding her hand, and she is dying. I know it won't be long now. Some few hours or perhaps days, at the very most. The family are standing outside the door. I can hear their harsh, whispering voices, for something fierce is going on out there, a major argument. The voices go to and fro, rising and falling, two sons, a daughter and some daughters-in-law. Suddenly, one of the sons opens the door and motions to me.

'My mother has agreed to certain changes in her will, Doctor. She decided on this earlier in the week, when we all met together, and just before she started going downhill. I wonder if you could just witness her signing the amended will. As an independent witness, as it were. It's all quite straightforward.'

I notice how he is staring straight past me, his voice hard but beginning to crumble at the edges. He carries the document into the stuffy room, folded so that I cannot see its contents – only the dotted lines where we will both sign: first her, then me. I see that he has already written in today's date. He looks towards the doorway.

'We've discussed it in full with her, Doctor, I can assure you. The three of us. She's agreed to all the changes. Haven't you, Mum?'

I say: 'I need to speak to her on her own. Completely on her own. To make *quite* sure that she does agree. That nothing's being done against her wishes, if you see what I mean. I'm sure you understand.'

I am surprised by the harshness of my own voice. Slowly, reluctantly, the son leaves the room, closing the door heavily behind him. I can hear him, or the others, leaning right against the door, almost breathing through the keyhole. I lean over her frail form, speaking clearly into her tiny, withered ear.

'Mrs Evans, your son says that you've agreed to certain changes in your will. Is that true? I don't need to know what they are. Only that you've agreed to them, and that you know what you've agreed to. Do you understand? Please tell me. It's very important that I'm sure that you know exactly what you're signing. And of your own free will. Do you understand what I'm saying?'

Outside the door, there is shuffling. A whispered argument has begun again, voices rising and falling. The old woman opens her eyes. Her voice is thin and faint. Like her body now, it is composed almost entirely of air. She nods, but there is the faintest trace of a smile on her toothless gums. 'I agree with them, Doctor, 'she says, 'Yes, I agree with all the changes. Every one of them. Everything changes, isn't that true?

I know just what I'm doing. And why I'm...' Her voice fades away, then she looks at me again in surprise. 'Everything changes...' she says again, and makes her unsteady mark on the paper.

I sign and leave the room, avoiding looking directly at any of them as they stand bunched around the doorway, staring in at the shadowy bed and at the document lying beside it.

It is a particularly icy Boxing Day, and I am on call for emergencies. With my small car skidding and sliding along the icy roads, I make my way to a house call. Shivering and clutching my bag, I trip and slither up the frozen garden path to the front door. Inside, the house is warm and stuffy, the air sour and hazy with tobacco smoke. A fire burns in the grate. As the mist clears from my glasses, I can see a big Christmas tree in one corner, festooned with multi-coloured lights and silver ornaments. Other silver ornaments and rows of gold-foil angels dangle from the ceiling. In another corner there is a high pile of opened presents and scrunched-up balls of torn wrapping paper. The whole family – parents, three or four teenage children, a few aunties and uncles – are gathered around the television set, holding cans of beer or bottles of Coke. For a moment they look up at me with puzzlement, then turn back to the game show on the telly. The audience has begun to scream. Someone on the show is about to win the Big Prize, but it's certainly not me – no one seems to be paying me any attention.

'I'm the doctor,' I say, loudly, 'The *doctor*. You told the receptionist you needed an urgent house call. You said that your daughter was ill, that she couldn't breathe properly. That's why I've come'.

The father drags his eyes slowly away from the screen and shrugs.

'Oh, that's Mary here,' he says, 'she's got a bad cold or something. Her nose is blocked. She's coughing a bit. Ain't you, love?' Sitting beside him Mary, 15 or so, shrugs. 'Suppose so,' she says.

I follow her to her bedroom, and examine her. The room is lined with posters of pop stars and other celebrities, young beardless men with thick lips and long eyelashes. A pile of small pink teddy bears lies beside the pillow.

There is nothing to be found. Nothing is really wrong with her. A minor respiratory infection, that's all. Outside, I can hear the snow beginning to throw itself violently against the window panes. I wonder if my car will start again in all this cold and damp. With difficulty, I only just manage to stop myself from strangling her with my stethoscope, and then getting to work on her father. But I say nothing. Nothing at all. We return to the lounge, and she resumes staring at the TV. Everyone ignores me. No one offers me coffee or a drink. In fact, no one says anything to me at all, as I stand awkwardly in the doorway. *Right*, I think. Still standing, I write out a prescription for cough medicine, paracetamol and a decongestant.

'I'm afraid you'll just have to get them for her,' I say, 'today. As you say, she's got a bad cold. As you say, she can't breathe properly through her nose. That's why you called me out, isn't that so? Now look, there's an emergency pharmacy in --. I think it's only about five or so miles from here. Not more than that. '

They stare up at me from the settee. Their faces have turned white as the blizzard outside.

'Merry Christmas!' I say and walk out, hunched against the driving snow.

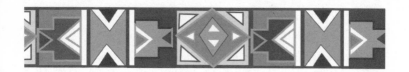

CHAPTER
12

An Autumn Leaf

V arsha watches the colours go by, jerking slowly past her on the moving river of grey rubber: canned fruit, breakfast cereals, frozen peas and ice-cream cartons, lettuce and celery and dark red apples, green peppers, bottles of orange juice, followed by blushing tomatoes and packets of brown bread. She watches them closely from behind her cash register. They are always the same, always in that same order of colours: green-yellow-red. And then at the end of the line: *brown.*

'Green-yellow-red-brown', she says to me, '*Now* do you understand?'

She wipes her eyes again and reaches forward. At the edge of my desk, the box of Kleenex is almost empty now. I don't know who needs them more by now, she or I. For a moment I stop writing and glance up again. Seated opposite me the tiny Indian woman in the creased brown sari is still hunched over in her chair like a question mark. And she is still staring down at the floor, her voice flat and paper-thin and sighing at the edges. There is a long grey plait hanging down her back, and the red *bindhi* on her forehead is almost lost among the deep cor-rugations there, but I notice that there is no wedding ring on her agitated fingers. Sitting besides her, heavily lipsticked and in tight sweater and jeans, her daughter translates haltingly from the Gujurati, her voice a tremulous echo of her mother's.

Suddenly Varsha breaks into English again.

'You know, Doctor, you know what it all means is that they want to ruin everything I have got. Everything I have in my life will go brown, you know. Brown! The curse they have given me will act against all the green, and turn it into yellow and red, and then into brown. Now you understand?'

But I understand nothing. Nothing. Nor do the shelves of medical textbooks in my bookcase, with their plump spines and confident golden lettering. Nor the rows of silver instruments, in the glass-fronted cabinet. None of us understands. On my desk, even the yellow daffodils in their vase are drooping with exhaustion, and I know how they feel. Glancing through the windows I can see down into the public park next door to the Medical Centre. The colours there are muted today, the trees leafless and skeletal under a low leaden sky. London in the late autumn. Already the air outside is damp, the grass soggy and brown with mud. I wish it were summer again. And I wish the beating of my heart would slow down a bit.

She begins to sob again, and now the daughter becomes mother, her hand circling the thin shaking shoulders, at first tentatively, but then more firmly.

'You know, Doctor, it means that if all the green in me goes – you know, if it dies and withers – then I will become not fertile. Not alive, you know. It's like a tree. Or a plant in the cold winter. The curse will destroy everything that I have got –'

The curse?

She tells me again that it had all begun several weeks ago, with yet another angry phone call from her former brother-in-law. Even though it had happened many years ago, she says that Rajinder is still bitter about the divorce. He blames her for it, and for the shame that it brought on them all.

'He says to me again,' she says, 'Rajinder says so to me again: "I will make sure that you never get the happiness again. Never!" Every time we speak together on the telephone, he says that to me.'

The next day, she says, her friend and next-door neighbour died unexpectedly of a heart attack. And then on the night of her friend's funeral, she had that dream. Tossing about in her bed, Varsha felt Rajinder's dog biting into her. She could feel its sharp teeth and the hot, panting slaver of its breath on her skin. Among the shifting moods and colours, she tried to pat it gently and to soothe it. 'I won't hurt you,' she said, again and again, 'I don't mean you any harm'. But in the morning, the marks of the dog's teeth were deep on her wrist, though only she could see them.

Some days later, coming home from the supermarket, she found three red roses lying on her bed. What were they doing there? She asked herself: did I buy them, or did someone else? But somehow she couldn't quite remember. Everything seemed confused. Gently she stroked their velvet petals. For a moment, she remembered how, also so gently, her husband had smiled at her on their wedding night as he had strewn handfuls of rose petals across their marital bed, before staining its sheets with tiny drops of her blood. But these particular roses were not scented messengers of love She knew that it was their thorns that were meant for her, not their petals. Wondering what they might mean, she remembered how in the dying days of her marriage, many years before, her husband had given her three red rose bushes to plant in their garden. From that moment onwards, she says, everything had seemed to go wrong. One piece of bad luck after another. ('Everything gone wrong, Doctor, just like now.'). When he finally left her, she had uprooted them and flung them angrily into the cellar. And now they were back again.

And then finally, a week before coming to see me, someone had entered her house while she was at work, and ransacked it.

'I think maybe my husband and his brother, they did it,' she says, 'because I think, maybe, they still have the keys to the front door.'

Among the missing items were her National Insurance card, a cheque book, her passport, her birth certificate, and some other official documents. Without them she feels obliterated, empty, confused. Someone has taken away her identity. She had called the police, and they advised her to change the front-door lock immediately. But they didn't seem at all interested in her story, especially when she told them in detail about the three red roses she'd found strewn across her bed – and those three unlucky rose plants in the garden, so many years before.

I page quickly through her medical notes, but already I know most of her story. Born in Uganda, to a family of comfortably off merchants living just outside Kampala until the dictator Idi Amin came to power, expelling all the Asians, rich and poor, Hindu and Muslim alike. Now in exile in England, after the death of her parents and the acrimonious divorce, she feels she has almost nothing. The four older children have married and moved far away. Now there is only this daughter, her supermarket job and the malevolent shadows of her ex-husband, now re-married, and his brother Rajinder, still living just around the corner. Even her sunny childhood memories of Africa are beginning to go, fading away like an old daguerreotype. Lonely in the cold grey drizzle of London, with its wet swishing roads and opaque sky, she lives in a city that feels both crowded and empty at the same time. As she speaks, I recognise that feeling and the pain that goes with it: the isolation, the sun-filled memories that live just behind your eyelids, the cultural double-vision that you develop. For I too am an immigrant to London, and I also was born in Africa, though down at its southernmost tip. The skies at the Cape of Good Hope are as deep and pellucid as those up in Uganda, an inverted ocean high above your head, and there too the African horizons seem to stretch everywhere and forever.

Listening to her, I have a sudden flash. I remember reading that in many cultures around the world Paradise is conceived of as a garden. Eden is always green, the colour of life, of foliage and food, and living plants. In arid lands especially, green has a special resonance. In the annual rebirth of living nature, fertility is always green. Green represents newness, hope, the freshness of spring set against the tired colours of the year's end. Yellow, red and brown are usually the colours of autumn, then of winter, the colours of decay and of dead and dying things. Now, nearing the end of this particular year, she sits in her dark brown sari opposite me, as thin and fragile as an autumn leaf. Her body so dry and brittle that I am afraid that if I speak too loudly to her, my breath could easily blow her away.

Deep within myself, two people are arguing fiercely – the young doctor and the anthropology graduate. It's a fierce debate, and I am the anxious referee. My medical books are of no use here, none at all. Fresh to family practice, I like to see myself as an 'expert' on cross-cultural medicine, as 'culturally-sensitive' to people from other backgrounds – unlike so many of my white-coated colleagues in hospitals who are more interested, it seems, in scans and printouts and fancy diagnostic machinery than in the real people that they deal with. I despised them at medical school, and I despise them now. It's the conceit of a very young doctor, fresh from a postgraduate degree in anthropology, to see myself as more than just a physician – as also a healer, an intellectual, a skilled social scientist. But there's also another reason. From medical school onwards and from my experience of growing up in a medical family, I have vowed never to medicalise the human condition, never casually to convert everyday human problems into medical diagnoses, and, in practice, always to try to use drugs sparingly with my patients, and only when really necessary. Above all, my vow is to try to treat medically what is medical, culturally what is cultural.

It doesn't help that, as the son of a psychiatrist, I also see myself (at least in those early days) as being strongly 'anti-psychiatric'. I have been heavily influenced by the writings of R.D. Laing, David Cooper, Thomas Szasz and other psychiatric heretics (not to mention the movie *One Flew Over the Cuckoo's Nest*) – all of whom saw madness as merely a normal person's response to an abnormal life, or an abnormal society. Often (particularly in those early days in practice) I also find myself being particularly critical of my medical colleagues, especially the psychiatrists, for confusing culture with pathology, for not understanding the obvious point that what may be 'normal' behaviour in one cultural group, may not be so in another; that 'mad' behaviour in one society, may be seen as 'bad' in another. And in clinical practice, they seem to miss so many of their patients' cultural cues, and thus fall into the trap of mistaking sadness for madness, human suffering for psychiatric syndromes – especially when that suffering is described by their patients in religious or supernatural terms: as due to Divine Punishment, say, or to witchcraft, voodoo or the Evil Eye. Or to a curse.

Despite this background scepticism, while Varsha and her daughter sit in front of me I can still feel my fingers creeping, of their own volition, towards my prescription pad. Even without consulting me, they have made their own decision. And I know, too, what would happen if they were to creep in the other direction, towards the telephone. I know well the likely denouement. For I have several times visited my patients in those big redbrick buildings, hidden behind high stone walls and tall trees. I have peered into the long fluorescent rooms smelling of urine and floor polish, at all those pale statues of trembling flesh frozen at intervals within them, standing quietly here and there, or shuffling stiffly in their old bathrobes among its long rooms and disinfected corridors – all those empty eyes and twitching faces, those sad irregular smiles gathered silently around the television set, under the watchful eyes of the burly male nurses in their half-length white coats.

It's also easy for me to imagine all those bespectacled strangers, perhaps some resembling my father, their faces frozen into benevolent masks, who would listen gravely to every detail of Varsha's story, her fears and dreams, her chaotic kaleidoscope of colours. And the curse. Yes, especially the curse. I think of all their bulging folders, the pages of notes that they would scribble about her, underlined with a colour symbolism of their own. How they would slowly nod their heads as she speaks. And how, eventually, they would probably label her as a 'paranoid schizophrenic', or perhaps just as someone with a 'depressive illness', a 'thought disorder' or 'paranoid ideation'. That big redbrick building would become another form of exile for her, another type of loneliness – cultural, as well as personal. I feel for her.

How would she cope, I wonder, with being asked regularly to 'share her feelings' with people she had never met before? Or with those other bespectacled strangers who would encourage her to develop something they called 'insight', to admit to them that, after all, she *was* cursed and possessed – but not by someone else, only by her own self and the malign demons of her own subconscious. I wonder how she would cope.

There is a sudden burst of Gujurati. Her daughter is staring closely at my face. 'Please, Doctor, please,' she says, 'Please don't send her to them. You know who I mean. My mother says that she would like to try something else first. Just for a week or two.'

For the first time, Varsha looks up from the worn carpet. Her eyes are quite red now, like two tiny berries embedded in her face. The pale skin is taut across her facial bones. I notice the faintest trace of a moustache on her trembling upper lip, and wonder if it was there when she first entered the room.

'Doctor,' she says slowly, 'Maybe I should just go to see a *vaid*, and ask him what is happening to me. What I should do. I have heard of a good one outside of London. In Luton.'

Vaids. I have read somewhere that there are several hundred of these Indian traditional healers in Britain, working among the south Asian communities. Practitioners of the ancient medical system of Ayurveda, derived from the Vedas, the Hindu holy books written in Sanskrit about 4000 years ago. Studying anthropology, I have read too about their complex views of health and illness, and how both are believed to be due to the subtle interplay and balance between different elements, especially between the *bhūtas*, the five basic elements of the universe – ether, wind, water, earth and fire – and the humours, and organs, that they form within the body. Apart from this, I know very little about these *vaids*, except that with their ancient wisdom and their holistic view of illness they should know how to deal with this type of situation better than any Western doctor. They will treat culturally what is obviously cultural. After all, they have had thousands of years' experience of doing just that.

'Can we please not wait some more time, Doctor,' says the daughter again, 'just a bit longer?'

'OK,' I say, though my voice is now as uncertain as her own. 'OK, if she wants to see him, she can. I can't stop her, but – '

Varsha nods vigorously, 'Yes,' she says, 'that would be good. *He* would understand me.'

I write out a prescription for an anti-depressant – a low dose. I tell her daughter to phone me immediately if anything new develops, any signs of worsening of her mother's mental state. I ask to see them both the following week. I escort her and her tiny pale mother over to the door.

'Oh by the way,' I hear myself calling out to Varsha, 'Eat lots and lots of greens. Anything green. Fresh fruits and salads and vegetables. Apples, lettuces, broccoli, spinach, anything. You look rather pale, and you're a vegetarian. So eat lots of them. You'll need them. They're really good for you.'

That night I sleep fitfully. My dreams are a confusion of many different colours. The images flow swiftly by: brown biting dogs, decomposing plants, dark thorns that prick me till I bleed. In the gaps of wakefulness, I wonder whether I have done the right thing. Is it ethical? Legal? Or have I made a terrible mistake? Perhaps her reactions are just the normal ones to her abnormal situation, with all its loneliness, loss and persecutions. Perhaps R.D. Laing was right. Or perhaps, like the malevolent husband in George Cukor's movie *Gaslight*, her ex-husband and his brother, or someone else, really are trying to trick her into thinking she is mad. Or maybe, after all, she really is psychotic.

I dream that someone in my dream is trying to tell me the answer, but somehow I cannot hear what they're trying to say.

It's a week later, and today Varsha is all alone sitting across the desk from me. Her voice is still flattened and sad, but the skin of her face less taut, her fingers less agitated.

'I did not see that *vaid* in Luton,' she says, shaking her head, 'he was away. Back in India. But I did go to see another one. Here in London. In Southall.'

'And…?' My pen hovers again in mid-air.

'Well, this *vaid* is very good. He says yes, I am right. My ex-husband and Rajinder *are* doing it to me. A curse, you know. And he is helping me to find out where they have put it.'

Tied on her right wrist, I notice a black thread. Later I learn that this is a *raksha*, one of the charms or amulets that some Indian folk healers give to their clients. She tells me how the *vaid* made his diagnosis – not by a stethoscope, an X-ray or an MRI scan, but by holding this black thread in his long fingers before he tied it onto her wrist. He then told her to close her eyes very tightly and prayed over her, asking her what she could see. And there, in the red velvety darkness behind her eyelids, she could see it clearly: her ex-husband putting a curse on her, inserting the spirits of several snakes into her body, one after the other, to cause her suffering and pain.

She closes her eyes for a moment. 'I can see how he puts a green snake inside of me, Doctor. And then a yellow snake. Then a red one. And then a brown snake spirit, all inside of me.'

'Snakes?'

'Yes, well, you know, the *vaid* says that the green snake sucks all the greenery out of me. The red snake is to suck my blood. The brown snake wants to kill my daughters and me, and turn everything brown. And the yellow snake is to destroy the gold.'

'The gold?'

'Yes, all the gold inside of me. All the treasure.'

For a moment I wonder what Sigmund Freud would have had to say about all this, about all those snakes entering her body, one after the other, consuming all of her hidden treasures. But this is London, well into the 20th century, not *fin-de-siècle* Vienna, and we are back to the colours again. Green-yellow-red-brown. And now gold.

Despite all of this, she seems to be recovering, though slowly. Her talks with the *vaid* appear to be helping her. She seems calmer. Sometimes, over the next few days, she even smiles a little. Several weeks later, I am celebrating the victory of anthropology over psychiatry when there's a sudden relapse. The colours are back. Some new 'messages' have appeared as coloured pieces of paper stuck onto road signs. She has even seen the date of her younger daughter's birthday written in red on a lamppost. On the bus to work, she has noticed a pink headband and a red-coloured bangle lying on the floor. And on a nearby seat, a black umbrella. That night she dreamt of the umbrella. 'It means I might become a widow,' she says, 'someone without shelter.' Right at the end of this dream, a broom appeared – small, brown, but large enough, she says, 'to sweep up the whole family'.

She is beginning to panic, and I am, too. I decide to give it just a few days more, no more than that, before making that final phone call.

But then only a day or so later, it finally happens. Quite unexpectedly, the sign that the *vaid* has long been waiting for …

Years before, Rajinder had given her a pet bird as a present, and she had kept it in a wire cage in her kitchen ever since. Now, while cleaning out the cage, the bird has suddenly flown out and disappeared through the open window, flapping its way to freedom. It all happened in a moment. Just like that. The *vaid* nodded gravely when he heard this story. He seemed to take it very seriously. He interrogated her closely about every detail, every tiny aspect of the event, exactly how it had happened, and when. Then finally he smiled in satisfaction.

'Yes, yes,' he said, 'Yes, yes, of course. That is just what I have been trying to do.'

He explained to her that by his magic he had managed to capture the evil spirit possessing her, then placed it invisibly inside her brother-in-law's dog, the one that had bitten her in the dream. Later he had carefully transferred it from Rajinder's dog into the bird, which has now flown away. In a series of steps, he said, he has finally freed her of the curse. It is all over now, he said.

'The *vaid* says he has now got rid of the curse,' she smiles, 'and now we can all of us sleep peacefully again!'

Months pass. I see her several times again in my office. She does look peaceful. Sitting upright in her chair, the folds of her bright emerald sari are rimmed in gold. Her face is still pale, but the *bindhi* glows more brightly now on the smooth skin of her forehead. Her voice is clear as she tells me that she is feeling much calmer these days, much easier. She is also sleeping better. She still sees the *vaid* regularly, and every week he says prayers for her. He has also given her a bottle of special water to drink, after praying over it for a long time.

In the supermarket, the groceries now move past her in a random kaleidoscope of colours. No more messages are hidden among the salads and the cellophane packets, the cereal boxes and the canned vegetables, as they flow swiftly out of sight on the grey river of rubber.

It's spring again. The days are lengthening, the parks of London ablaze with new colour, beds of roses, geraniums, daffodils and pansies. One warm evening I am sitting in a restaurant with my friend, a psychiatrist. He comes originally from India.

'So why did she get better?' I ask him, ''Why did she recover?'

He shakes his head. He frowns, then shakes it again.

'You know,' he says, 'I recognise only small, tiny bits of her story, but not the rest of it. Mostly it's unfamiliar to me.'

He says that during her breakdown she seems to have blended a few traditional Indian images with her own more idiosyncratic fantasies, into a personalised landscape of persecution and fear.

'In fact, I think the whole story is hardly cultural at all,' he says, 'Not at all. I think it's just straight psychiatric.'

'Yes, but at least it shows that traditional healing works,' I say, 'that non-Western forms of healing such as Ayurveda actually work. Whether by suggestion or whatever. And that you don't always have to rely on the shrinks when people get mentally ill. And on their drugs and their shock therapy, their locked wards, and all the rest. In the end it was the *vaid* that had the answer, not them. After all, those *vaids* have had about four thousand years to perfect their skills.'

My friend looks at me strangely.

'Yes, it is odd,' he says frowning, 'that she got better. Especially since she's never even *seen* a *vaid*.'

For a long while we sit in silence. I wait for my heart to stop beating so violently, and for my breathing to slow down to normal again.

'Why, what do you mean? Of course she's seen one. What about the man she saw in Southall?'

'Oh no, no, no, he's not a real *vaid* at all,' he says, 'I can assure you of that. In fact, I wonder how she found him. Not the real thing at all, probably just some *jadoo-tona wallah*. You know, they're the sort of faith healer or magico-religious type of practitioner that you find in the little villages back in India. They deal with curses, Evil Eye and all that sort of thing. They're very popular among the simple, superstitious people, you know, but they're not qualified. Not in real Ayurveda. No, no, this chap is obviously a fake. A quack. Definitely not a real *vaid* at all.'

'So why did she get better, then?'

My friend shrugs. 'Who knows?' he says, 'Maybe she didn't really. I mean, not in the long-term. In any case –'

Suddenly he rises to his feet. 'Look,' he says, 'it's still light. Let's forget about all this shop talk and go for a walk in the park. Even this late, you still catch the scent of all those new spring flowers out there. The park is full of them ...'

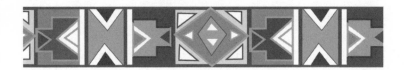

CHAPTER
13

The Illusion of Doubles

The page is embossed at the top with the logo and name of the local mental hospital. The paper feels thick and official. It's a report from one of the senior psychiatrists at the hospital, written in his arcane professional dialect. The letter provides cold clinical subtitles to this particular story of human anguish I had witnessed at its conclusion. As I read it, I remember how Mrs P had sat on the settee in her sitting room with that insouciant smile, trembling slightly ('regards herself as completely normal, and has absolutely no insight into her illness'); how she had puffed her way through a full packet of Gauloise ('smoked cigarettes in a hectic and chaotic fashion'); how, at one stage, she had got up and moved around the room, shifting magazines and newspapers on a sideboard from one pile to another ('engaged in irrelevant displacement activity'). Right at the foot of his report, and heavily underlined, is the psychiatrist's final diagnosis – two unfamiliar words that will be branded on her forever, like a mark of Cain: '*Capgras Syndrome*'.

The psychiatrist's letter recalls a visit to Mrs P's house several weeks before. The house is in one of those suburbs of small near-identical houses that you find in towns all over southern England, each with its own tiny garden, its own neatly trimmed hedge or little white wall – the sort of suburb that you drive through without even noticing it. But inside this particular house, the atmosphere is charged, and very unusual. Something brittle and volatile is in the air, almost as if we have wandered into the very centre of an electrical storm. There are four of us standing in the entrance hall: the psychiatrist, the social worker, and two very young doctors – one of whom is me.

The décor inside the house is almost identical to many of the other houses in the street and in others elsewhere in the city – the same thick pile carpets and floral curtains, the same cream wallpaper. On the walls framed mirrors, several bright prints of landscapes or crying clowns. On the mantelpiece, among crowds of tiny porcelain figurines, is a row of family photographs in imitation gilt frames. There's the standard suite of chintz, with modest settee and comfortable armchairs, and, resting on those familiar tables of glass and stainless steel, the familiar vases of flowers, real or imitation, while in the windows the same lace curtains flap away like petticoats. Even the warm, slightly chemical air of the room seems familiar, with its distinctive incense of suburbia: furniture polish, air freshener and detergents.

Sitting on the settee, tremulous and thin, Mrs P is puffing away at a cigarette. Already the ashtray in front of her is overflowing. Her dark hair, streaked with grey, is drawn back in haphazard strands and tied at the back of her head. Under her pale forehead, corrugated with frowns, the eyes are hooded and darting. She wears no make-up. Something about her fine tremor seems to give her an insubstantial air, like the hot shimmer of a desert mirage.

Mr P, seated besides her, is in his mid-sixties or so, short and stocky, with a broad neck and rectangular face, and a corona of wiry grey hair that circles his bald head like icy clouds on a mountain top. He has the big, hairy, practical hands of a builder or a farmer. Now he sits uneasily, mouth tightly closed. He has the look of a man only just holding something inside himself: a great subterranean anger, perhaps. They have no children.

The psychiatrist sits down beside her, while the rest of us seat ourselves down around the room, spectators of this deadly drama. In the background I can hear the voices of two or three women, talking softly in the kitchen. Soon one of them appears, a neighbour or a friend or relative, eyes bloodshot and swollen, carrying a little tea tray, which she lays down before Mrs P.

Mrs P puts down her cigarette and lifts up the teapot. She pours the hot liquid into our cups, which clatter in their saucers. We are all waiting. Eventually she puts down the teapot, stubs out her cigarette, and begins her story. It all started, she says, with that thin watery fluid that has recently begun to pour out of the top of her head. In the past week or so, it has happened to her twice already. And each time, just before it happened, her skull had unexpectedly 'opened up' to let the fluid flow out.

As she reaches forward to hand us our cups of tea, I find myself taking a deeper breath, for right on the top of her scalp a circular patch has been shaved – a neatly trimmed bald area, right at the very crown of her head, like a crop circle or the spoor of a UFO burnt into a cornfield.

I am still staring at it as she goes on to describe those invisible currents of 'electricity' – the ones that have begun to leak from the walls, the television set and the cooker in the kitchen – and how they have influenced her thoughts and infiltrated her dreams. How they send tingles up and down her body whenever she walks past a plug socket in the wall, even when it's been switched off. And how, for several weeks now, these currents have forced her to sleep out in the garden shed at night, swaddled like a frightened fetus in the depths of a sleeping-bag.

Outside, through the large glass doors, I can see that the rectangular lawn is so tightly mown that it resembles a green carpet, newly shampooed. Surrounding it are orderly ranks of disciplined flowers. On the fence, a few wild red roses have been tightly tied to their trellises, with any dissident branches carefully pruned away. At the very bottom of the garden you can just make out a little wooden garden shed of brown clapboard, with a small door and double windows: a tiny pastiche of an English country cottage.

But it's not just her story that holds our bodies rigid at the edges of our chairs, like manikins in a wax museum, or even the stifled sounds of sobbing from the kitchen. No, it's the odd way that she speaks about her husband, avoiding his name, referring to him always as 'this man'.

On the settee beside her, 'this man' shifts uneasily. Suddenly he jumps to his feet and walks heavily out of the room. At the door he stops, looks back at us, then disappears, shaking his head. As soon as he's gone, she turns towards us, eyes narrowed, her voice soft and sideways: 'Did you see the man's legs?' she asks, 'Did you notice the way that he crossed them when he was sitting down here, one over the other? The left one over the right – like this. Not the other way round, like the real one always used to do. What did I tell you?'

Sips of tea are burning my throat, like droplets of acid. She draws diagrams in the air with trembling fingertips.

'It's from little signs just like that that I know what's happening,' she says, 'That I know that he's not the real one. Not the real John. A wife always knows her husband well, isn't that so? And I don't know who this man is, though I must say he does look quite a lot like John. But he's someone else, pretending to be my husband. Last week I tried to tell him about all the electricity from the walls, and how it's hurting my body, really hurting me, but he said that he didn't understand a word I was saying. Not a word. So how can he possibly be the *real* John?'

On the glass table, the cups of tea are still untouched, wrinkled membranes forming across their surfaces. Scribbling in his notebook, the psychiatrist asks her several more questions, then puts down his pen and glances towards us. He has moved to centre stage; the spotlight is on him now. An ambiguous sigh has entered his voice now; it is full of sadness. He tells her that he is very worried about her, that she is not well. He says he understands what is happening to her and what she has been telling us, and how frightening it must be for her. He wants to help her, in any way he can, and to take her away from all that electricity and those other things. For only a short time, he promises. Enough time for a 'few tests' to be carried out. He says that she definitely needs to be given some 'medicines' in the hospital, which will make her feel much better. And she needs them *soon*. Today. In fact, right now. He sighs again, but already something has begun to harden and solidify in the air around him:

'I hope, of course, that you will agree to come in voluntarily,' he says, 'but if that is not possible, then I'm afraid that I…'

I find myself staring into the far corner of the room while the others scribble away. A pile of paperback books lie neatly stacked there beside the big television set, containing so many human stories all locked up inside those thin rectangular shapes – each the flat container of all the colour, movement and emotion of a particular life, whether real or fictitious. Just as Mrs P herself will soon be contained, compressed, turned into the pages of a bulging psychiatric file. Hunched over in her chair, the social worker writes busily in the wad of papers scattered across her lap.

Mrs P is still vainly refusing. 'But I'm all right, Doctor', she is saying, over and over again, 'I'm fine myself, I'm OK. There's nothing wrong with me. It's this man who is doing this to me. You can see what he's doing, can't you? All that electricity that he's using. He's the one who needs you, not me.'

For a split-second I find myself wondering. Perhaps, after all, she is right, for there is something rather odd about her husband as he stands silently in the doorway. I notice that now he has begun to tremble at the edges too as if, like his wife, he has gradually metamorphosed into something less sure, less substantial.

Suddenly her head darts forward again, and as she does so the hair rises at the back of my neck. Her voice is low and confidential, eyes darting quickly from side to side, face contracted into a grimace of terror. She is whispering so low now that we can hardly hear her:

'If I ever leave this house,' she says softly, 'if I ever go into hospital, you know what will happen then, don't you?'

We lean forward to catch her fading voice.

'As soon as I leave here,' she says, 'he will replace me with another woman. An exact copy of myself. '

In 1923 two French psychiatrists, Dr Capgras and Dr Reboul-Lachaux, writing in the *Bulletine de la Société Clinique de Médecine Mentale*, described a new syndrome which they called *l'illusion de sosies* ('The illusion of doubles'). Now it's called *Capgras syndrome*. Apparently more common in men than in women, it is often a symptom of grave mental illness, a severe type of delusion. Usually the victims believe that someone close to them – a spouse, parent, child or neighbour – has been replaced by an evil impostor. Often the impostor appears to be an exact replica of the original, with every wart, wrinkle and gesture cleverly reproduced. To achieve this, the doubles have been endlessly cunning. They have in many cases used wigs, masks, make-up, costumes, elaborate disguises or even expensive plastic surgery, to alter their appearance. But there are always clues, tiny, subtle clues, which only the victim can detect.

In some of the cases, the evil double is believed to have secretly abducted or even murdered the original. In others, the doubles themselves proliferate, in an act of malevolent mass production, into a whole crowd of identical impostors. And sometimes – perhaps most terrifying of all – the victims fear that, like Mr Golyadkin in Dostoyevsky's *The Double*, they themselves have been duplicated, and are now being impersonated by a double.

Since 1923 hundreds more cases of the syndrome have been identified by psychiatrists. Their reports have been published in dozens of journals, suggesting a veritable epidemic of duplications, a plague of imitations – but especially in the industrialised countries of Western Europe and North America.

Thinking back on her now, many decades later, I realise that for me Mrs P's greatest fear is a curious echo of Dostoyevsky's short, but haunting novel. In *The Double* a certain Mr Golyadkin, a minor civil servant in St Petersburg, comes home one evening to find a stranger waiting for him at the entrance to his apartment building. The man follows him up the stairs, enters his apartment, and then without explanation sits down confidently upon his bed. With horror, Golyadkin realises who he is: 'Mr Golyadkin's nocturnal acquaintance was none other than himself, Mr Golyadkin himself, another Mr Golyadkin, but exactly the same as himself, in short, in every respect what is called a double.' The stranger sitting on his bed is 'of the same height and build, dressed in the same way and with the same bald patch – in short, nothing, absolutely nothing was lacking to complete the resemblance.' The story is true gothic horror, a literary precognition of Capgras syndrome. For the double is sly and cunning, and gradually insinuates himself into Goldyadkin's life, usurping his job, his friends, and the woman he loves. Slowly Golyadkin slips into madness, the very existence of the double challenging his own sense of authenticity. It's as if he himself has become a counterfeit, instead of the other. At times he becomes 'like a man who for want of his own clothes is wearing someone else's.' In his final, thrashing nightmares, Golyadkin dreams of even more duplications, of 'a terrible multitude of perfect replicas.'

Rare though it is, Capgras syndrome has always seemed to me to be more than just a severe mental illness. Perhaps, in symbolic terms, it tells us a different, much deeper story. In the decades since I met her, I have often wondered whether poor Mrs P was actually quite as mentally disturbed as she seemed to be, or as the psychiatrist thought she was. And I have wondered whether, like some fragile and over-sensitive barometer, she had actually picked up some crucial aspects of the *zeitgeist*, the cultural atmosphere of our time – and then been crushed by the contradictions within it.

For like her, we all now live in a world of confusion, a world of copies and mass-production, in which every day millions of identical objects and images are being churned out: matching clothes and identical cars; multiple copies of books, magazines, cosmetics and lifestyles; 'chains' of near-identical McDonald's or hotels like the Hilton in every city; and the same face smiling at us from millions of newspapers or television screens. It's a world of fads and facsimiles, of fashions that sweep in waves through the community like high-priced plagues. Images of ourselves can now be multiplied endlessly by photography, videos, the Internet and the Xerox machine – and will soon be reproduced, even more accurately, by genetic cloning. Modern society has taken the cult of the copy further than ever before: from mass-produced everyday objects to all the imitation Elvis Presleys and the endless crowds of wannabe Madonnas or Marilyn Monroes.

Duplication and imitation – and the uneasiness they cause – are themes often reflected in popular culture, from movies like *Invasion of the Body Snatchers* or *The Stepford Wives*, to the repetitive images of Andy Warhol. They occur also in literature, as in Jorge Luis Borges's enigmatic parable *Borges and I*, about his problems with his own double: 'the other one, the one called Borges'. Gradually, like Mr Golyadkin's double, this evil impostor has taken over and subdued Borges's own life, till now he can no longer escape its clutches.

'Thus my life is a flight,' he writes, 'and I lose everything and everything belongs to oblivion, or to him.'

But then wryly concludes: 'I don't know which of us has written this page.'

In his essay *Travels in Hyperreality*, Umberto Eco notes another curious phenomenon of contemporary culture, especially in the United States. Travelling across that country, he visits innumerable theme parks and wax museums, historical tableaux and dioramas. In city after city he encounters 'exact replicas' of the celebrated art treasures of Europe: *The Last Supper*, the *Mona Lisa*, the *Venus de Milo*, the *palazzi* of Venice, and many others.

Touring these multiple museums, Eco describes how in these displays of American culture 'the authenticity is visual, not historical'.

'There is a constant in the average American imagination and taste for which the past must be preserved and celebrated in full-scale authentic copy, a philosophy of immortality as duplication'. The New World has reincarnated many of the cultural icons of Europe, in the form of 'authentic copies'. But there is one important difference. For Eco, many of these replicas seem somehow more 'real' to him – certainly cleaner, clearer and more accessible – than their originals back in Europe. As in *The Double* – or in Capgras syndrome – in the growing hallucinatory confusion between copy and original, the replica actually aims to be the thing, to become its perfect double, and thus to replace it. 'The American imagination demands the real thing,' writes Eco, 'and, to attain it, must fabricate the absolute fake'. He calls this phenomenon: 'hyperreality'.

Returning to Mrs P – weeping on her settee as she waits for the stern ambulance-men to come to take her away – I am still left wondering today whether she was a victim of this modern hyperreality, this pervasive confusion of images, of the constant blurring of boundaries between fiction and reality created by the media and by our consumerist culture. Or whether, she just symbolises for me something that is happening to all of us, though in a milder form, trapped as we are within that intrinsic fault-line of modern society: the basic contradiction between the cult of Individuality – and that of mass production.

Mrs P's anguish, her predicament, reaches forward to touch me, even after all these years. And it serves also to illustrate to me why – in the age of the fake, the exact facsimile, the clone and the mass-produced double – the modern self is so fragile, and so prone to existential anxiety and breakdown.

And why Golyadkin's anguished cry, near the end of Dostoyevsky's novel, as he slips deeper and deeper into the abyss of madness – 'Either you or I, one or the other, but both of us together is impossible!' – could be taken as one of the cries of this modern Age.

What I would call, the *Age of Capgras*.

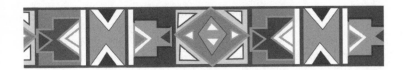

CHAPTER
14

Boundaries

Mr G is a heavy smoker, with yellowed fingertips and a deep, cavernous cough. The more he smokes, the more ill he gets: bronchitis, pneumonia, emphysema, a collapsed lung. And now his heart is beginning to pack up, and lung cancer waits in the wings. And yet he refuses to stop. And so do I, for every time I see him I plead with him once again to give up smoking.

'You'll kill yourself!' I cry out, again and again, 'You'll kill yourself if you carry on smoking. For the sake of your health, *stop!*'

And each time Mr G gives the same answer, and smiles at me in the same, insouciant way.

'*Yes, but...* ' he replies, and then carries on smoking.

Year after year I plead, give more advice, offer more statistics.

'Yes, but...' he says again, 'Yes, but ....'.

The game goes on for years, an exhausting game of ping-pong in which my advice flies in one direction across the desk and 'Yes, buts' come back in the other. It's a game in which I am always the loser, for after every match it is he who leaves the room, smiling and relaxed, to light up another fag as soon as he gets outside, while I am the one left slumped in my chair, exhausted, defeated.

I have known hundreds of Mr Gs (and Mrs Gs) in my clinical practice, and for many years they all had that same effect upon me. Whether smoking, drinking or harming themselves in another way, it was always the same. Faced with their obduracy it is I who collapse, not they. Maybe it's all because of my father's early death, after years of heavy smoking. Or maybe it's just me, losing sight of where I end and where they begin. A problem of boundaries.

One day, after much thought, I finally change the game.

'Mr G,' I say, 'as I've told you many times in the past, smoking so much is dangerous. It's going to kill you. You must give it up.'

I can see his lips forming, with pleasure, his usual reply, but I won't let him begin.

'You know all the dangers,' I say, 'You know all the diseases that smoking can cause you – cancer, heart disease and all the rest – don't you?'

He nods, uncertainly.

'Right,' I say, 'now its up to you to stop. I really can't make you stop, because…' – and then I administer the *coup de grace* – 'because, after all, it's *your* body that will get ill, *not mine!*'

Mr G falls back in his chair with shock. He looks baffled, pale, disappointed. He's been looking forward to a good game, and now it's as if I have unexpectedly leaned across the desk, seized the ping-pong bat out of his hand, and smashed it across his head. And then, for good measure, jammed the little white ball into his mouth and made him swallow it.

He leaves, muttering. Obviously I am a bad doctor. Obviously I don't care. And obviously he will soon go elsewhere. But meanwhile, it is I who sit back comfortably in my chair and give a deep sigh of contentment. The score? Twenty-love. To me.

To celebrate, I almost feel like lighting up a fag.

Until that moment, there had been a deep collusion between Mr G and myself, a *folie à deux*. I treated him, but in a way I was also treating myself, my own anxieties about him and about other things. This roundabout way of cure is one of the occupational diseases of the doctor, part of our *déformation professionelle*. It's been called 'the need to be needed'. It's often the reason why people go into medicine in the first place. And in some ways, it makes us particularly vulnerable, especially to patients' ungratefulness or to feelings of rejection.

But blurred boundaries are not just the doctor's problem. In family practice especially there are also many patients who, over the years, somehow absorb their doctor into their own self-image: as a helpful and extra organ, a prosthetic limb, a crutch. Sometimes it can go much further than that. In her book *Theatres of the Body*, the psychoanalyst Joyce McDougall describes the extreme case of Georgette, one of her clients, someone who at times 'did not truly distinguish between my body and hers, nor between our personal identities'. One year, when she sees McDougall come back tanned from her vacation, Georgette cries out in horror:

'What have you done to my face? My face is hurting badly.'

And each time her analyst goes away on vacation, Georgette breaks out in a red, raw rash all over her body. It's almost as if she'd been 'flayed alive', her epidermis ripped right off her. And one day, after passing McDougall's husband on her way in, she remarks:

'A nice surprise. I just met *our* husband in the street.'

Georgette and Mr G are obviously extreme examples, but in real-life medical practice doctors and patients can often dissolve into one another over many years, losing sight of where the one ends and the other begins. In some cases it can be a damaging process for both, containing within it the seeds of burnout for the one and deep dependency for the other. Freeing oneself from this situation means, among other things, dissolving the *folie à deux* between doctor and patient. It means re-establishing firm boundaries. And like the shaman or the psychoanalyst, it also means the doctor confronting, and then mastering, the doctor's own inner demons, not only the personal demons, but also those demons specific to the practice of medicine: the fear of making a mistake; the fear of missing a diagnosis; the fear of the closeness of death; and the fear of crossing the boundaries between Them and Us, and thereby entering too deeply into the Land of the Sick. And sometimes, allied with all of these fears, there are feelings of helplessness uncomfortably twinned with those of omnipotence.

Controlling all these internal demons can be an exhausting process. But for many patients, the visible exhaustion of their doctor is not the sign of a bad or a burnt-out physician. On the contrary, it's the sign of a good one. In his book *The Healer's Art*, for example, the New York physician Eric J. Cassell describes how at times, when he's feeling rested and 'fresh as a daisy', many of his patients tell him how totally exhausted he looks, how hard he must be working, how little sleep he must getting. At first Cassell wonders what they mean by these remarks. He decides that what is really being said here, is that 'fatigue is the real hallmark of the profession, because the struggle of the doctors is with death'.

In mythological terms, it's the exhaustion of the archetypal hero or heroine, fresh from their daily battle with the cosmic forces of Disease and Death. Like the shaman, he has to confront these evil forces and defeat them. It's an eternal battle, one that must continue for every day of the doctor's working life.

But there are other reasons for this exhaustion. 'One of the reasons that many physicians feel drained by their work' writes the cancer specialist Rachel Naomi Remen, 'is that they do not know how to make an opening to receive anything from their patients. The way we were trained, receiving is considered unprofessional. The way most of us were raised, receiving is considered a weakness.'

Old Dr Q, cynical and battle-hardened after forty years in family practice, would certainly not agree with her. He believes in very firm boundaries.

'If there's one thing much worse than turning a friend into a patient,' he warns me sternly, 'it's turning a patient into a friend!'

Even though she's not become a friend, and never will be, I think I have turned Mrs R into a sort of diagnostic test. Somehow, she's become a sensitive barometer of my own internal emotional state. More than most patients I know, she can reveal to me the state of my own boundaries, how needy I have become, how porous, how close to emotional burnout. Now she sits across the desk from me, her oval face smiling under its halo of white hair. Her expression, as usual, is soft and concerned. She is peering at me closely, leaning forward. And, as usual, she replies to my greeting with:

'But how are *you* feeling today, Doctor?'

Then always: 'You look very tired today, Doctor. Is everything OK? Are you sure? You really must be working very hard. You doctors work so hard, and no one really takes any notice, do they?' And then adds:

'No one appreciates what you do for them. People are *so* ungrateful to their doctors these days, don't you think?'

I nod in grateful agreement. With Mrs R in the room, I can feel myself beginning to relax after a long, hard day, to drop my guard. But already it's much too late.

Each time I see her, a warm feeling flows across the desk towards me. She is so concerned, so understanding, and so appreciative. What a change, I think. A consultation with her is like a jacuzzi in warm treacle, languid and deeply relaxing. And each time she leaves the room, I am left thinking: Yes, but why did she actually come in to see me? And each time, I can hardly remember, for it's as if she has lulled me into a deep, relaxed sleep, full of pleasant and unexpected dreams.

Usually it's only when she's already halfway out the door, and I have jolted awake, that I sometimes catch a glimpse of the prescription that she's clutching – written in my own handwriting – and can then remember why she actually came in to see me. And each time I warn myself to be more cautious, more alert with her next time. But that next time, particularly if I'm feeling bruised or burnt out (and she always senses if I am), and she returns with her sympathy and flowers, her chocolates and home-made jam, and her warm treacly voice, I find that all I want to do is to relax, to rest my tired head gratefully on her soft, scented shoulder. And soon I am fast asleep again.

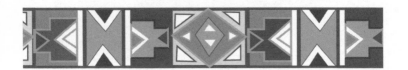

CHAPTER
15

Prescriptions

'Writing prescriptions is easy, but coming to an understanding with people is hard.'

Franz Kafka, *A Country Doctor*

John is a bitter man. He is well over sixty, and he feels a failure. All his big hopes and his big ambitions have turned to ashes, one after another. There seems to be nothing left of them now. His businesses have failed one by one, his plans collapsed. Now all that remains to see is this small man, bitter and brooding, with large debts and vanishing hair, and all the inner ulceration of defeated dreams. His wife Amanda is deeply unhappy, too, but in a very different way. She is loud and indignant, and somehow always seems to fill my room. She is like a large balloon filled with angry helium, floating somewhere high above the carpet, expanding with every moment until she occupies every corner and crevice of the room, and always ready to burst.

John and Amanda have a 'chemical marriage'. I call it that, because what glues them together is not just love. It is also chemicals. He takes regular tranquillisers, and she is always on anti-depressants. He takes a nightly sleeping tablet or two, and so does she. And both of them take more than the occasional drink in order, they say, 'to steady the nerves'.

They have been taking these chemicals for many years now, and every attempt to wean them off has failed. Many doctors (including myself) have tried and tried, and counsellors too, but each time one of them reduces their tablets, their relationship begins to fall apart. Without these powerful chemicals in their bloodstreams, they are quite unable to deal with her rage, his irritability, her hysterical weeping, his anxieties and her fears, as well as the irritable consequences of their shared insomnia.

John and Amanda are not that unusual in family practice. I've met scores of people like them over the years. But they always put their doctor in an awful dilemma, for without those drugs, poured daily down their throats, their marriages would undoubtedly explode. So that is the choice the doctor is often left with: either to put money into the pockets of the pharmaceutical industry, or else into those of the divorce lawyers. It's a hellish choice, but I know which one of these two I reluctantly prefer. It's a long time since I believed in what someone in the 1960s called 'pharmacological Calvinism': the notion that all drugs that improve your mood were bad, for they somehow make you less authentic and stunted your spiritual growth. No gain without pain, they always used to say. But sadly, in practice this often doesn't work – at least, not for people like John and Amanda.

Gladys is superstitious. She's a worshipper of the little gods, the gods of lotteries and luck, the gods of traffic jams and parking places, the one's to whom you pray for nice weather for a particular picnic, or for finding just the right sort of dress for that Christmas party, at just the right sort of price. Gladys relies on these small, personal gods to help her with the small, personal problems of her daily life.

She is elderly and unhappy. Except for her cat, she lives alone. She is often lonely. These days she believes especially in those tiny, circular gods that her doctors have prescribed for her, the one's they call tranquillisers. For her, these little round things have a powerful, talismanic quality. Even their minute size underlies the enormous healing energies condensed within them. She always keeps them in a small gold box on her dresser, its lid inlaid with mother-of-pearl.

Prozac is her best friend these days, Mogadon her night time lover.

In the past, she was married to Valium. Gladys speaks about them to her doctor almost as if they were people: a good friend, a companion, a spouse.

'I just couldn't get through the day without them', she says, 'I need them with me. They help me get through the day.'

'And without them?'

'Without them, Doctor,' she replies, 'I simply couldn't function. I couldn't sleep, I'd become withdrawn, I'd just cry all the time.'

'And what would happen then?'

'Then I'd probably die,' she says, ' Or just go completely mad.'

Most doctors have met many people like Gladys: sad, lonely people who feed chemicals to their loneliness to keep it at bay, who see these drugs as a sort of 'food' without which they feel they couldn't survive. They're different from John and Amanda, whose drugs are more the 'fuel' of their lives, something to make the worn-out engine of their marriage continue to run smoothly. But both are part of the same modern idea, the illusion of the 'pharmatocopia': that medicine can create (thanks to pharmacology) a world free of pain and unhappiness, one where, as with the *soma* in Aldous Huxley's *Brave New World*, there's a pill for every personal problem – and for every form of unhappiness. Today, in our rushed, competitive society, the pharmaceutical industry is making a lot of money out of pushing the contemporary formula, *a la* Aldous Huxley:

Person + Chemical = Happy Person.

Many doctors I know also have 'chemical marriages', not with their spouses usually, but with their patients – marriages in which doctor and patient are glued together by regular prescriptions from one to the other, whether for tranquillisers, heart drugs, blood pressure tablets or anything else. It's a type of dependency that the doctor needs to be aware of and, if possible, to fight. In some cases, it's the actual prescription, rather than the drugs themselves, that is the real bond between doctor and patient. Apparently in Britain many people don't even 'cash in' their prescriptions to the pharmacy, to collect their drugs. For many people, these tiny rectangular pieces of paper are more like symbolic contracts between doctor and patient: the patient's name written at the top of the paper, the doctor's name at the bottom, the two of them joined together by the scrawled name of the drug in-between. Taken home, they can be proudly displayed to the family as a badge of illness, a magnet for sympathy, a tangible token of the doctor's love – or even carried around for days in a pocket or handbag, as a healing talisman in their own right.

Just look at this big pile of glossy pamphlets sent to me by various pharmaceutical companies. There's a dozen of them lying on my desk. One advertises a new antidepressant tablet. It shows not the portrait of an unhappy person, but only a brightly coloured painting of his brain. Another, promoting an anti-arthritic drug, shows only an ankle and a hand, with all their joints swollen and red, but again no person. While a third, for a cardiac drug, shows a heart, all red and romantic – but also without any person attached to it. Like so many other such adverts in medical journals these days, they show only the diseased organ and of course the drug, not the patient. It's a way of thinking that has been called 'reductionism': reducing all the complexity of a situation, down to its very simplest elements – but, in the process, distorting it. In this case, it means reducing the complex idea of human suffering down to the disease of a particular organ. In medicine, it's a way of making (probably not consciously) disease more easily manageable, more containable, even if it makes it less human in the process.

Increasingly, the pharmaceutical companies want me to write pre-scriptions in order to solemnise some intimate, symbiotic relationship between their particular drug and a particular body part, or between the drug and a specific microbe or disease process. In fact, they want me to officiate at a series of chemical marriages. And although I always try to resist them as best I can, the pharmaceutical salesmen can be very persuasive, especially when it comes to antibiotics.

In a famous speech in 1906, the scientist Paul Ehrlich expressed the hope that one day, medicines 'able to exert their final action exclusive-ly on the parasite harboured within the organism would represent, so to speak, magic bullets which seek their target of their own accord.' Although the contemporary image is now less that of a bullet, and more of a laser-guided missile or 'smart bomb', many antibiotics are still marketed in the form of a bullet-shaped capsule, as a magic mis-sile made of gelatine. Even though Louis Pasteur himself once remarked that 'the microbe is nothing, the terrain, everything', adverts for antibiotics still often ignore the fact that it's people who have infections – and not the other way round: infected people who live in families, who have jobs, who dream and desire, who have deadlines to meet. Real people. Commonly these adverts portray a ruthless one-to-one battle deep within the body: not between a human being, his or her daily life, and a particular disease process, but merely a battle between a drug and a microbe. A deadly contest, portrayed in vivid Technicolor, as tiny hero and tiny villain, united by a prescription, are locked together in mortal combat.

The colourful world of the pharmaceutical advert is a fantasy world, one of the many fantasies spawned by modern techno-medicine. It's an abstract, microscopic, pared-down world, freed of all the ambiguities and uncertainties of the human condition. But sadly, some doctors today seem to prefer it to the real thing.

Warren is bent over, sweating, grunting with his back pain. He even finds it difficult to climb onto my examination couch. His back is in spasm, he says, and it's so painful that he can hardly move. He cries out 'Oh! Oh! Oh! Oh!' with every movement, or sometimes 'No! No! No! No!' when I try to examine him. He's rigid, wracked with pain. And that is why his cure, when it comes shortly afterwards, is so miraculous and so unexpected. For after a brief examination, some sympathetic words, a prescription for painkillers and a medical certificate entitling him to miss work for another two weeks, he is cured. Completely. Just look out of the window now, only a few moments later, and you'll see what I mean. Just after he's limped so painfully out of my room and staggered slowly down the stairs, I can see him striding across the park next door. Sometimes he breaks into a playful jump, sometimes he bends over nonchalantly to pick a flower. Sometimes he even kicks at a passing football. His movements are free now and fluent as a bird's. He looks happy. It's a miracle cure, no doubt of that. From my window I can see that he's clutching something white in his hand. Is it his medical certificate, the one that will pay him to stay off work for a week or two? Or is it rather his prescription, the one that he'll soon wave in his wife's sceptical face as he limps slowly, painfully through the front door of his home?

As Warren skips out of sight, I slap myself on the back. Once again,

I compliment myself on my healing powers and on the extraordinary, almost mystical power of my signature. Combined with it, the effects of those little scraps of paper are truly magical!

Suddenly there's a sound from behind me. Someone is clearing her throat. I turn away from the window overlooking the park and look around me. There's an elderly man and a woman there, still sitting across from my desk, and both of them are smiling up at me.

'Thanks, Doctor,' says Amanda, putting the two prescriptions carefully into her handbag, while John nods in grateful agreement, 'I really don't know what we'd do without you.'

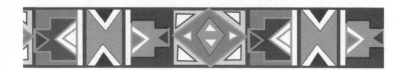

CHAPTER
16

Membranes

Often it's the very first lesson you learn in medical practice, sometimes on the first day – the lesson that the membrane between life and death is thin and transparent, and so easily crossed. Once learned, it is never forgotten.

One morning at the Medical Centre, a young man, full of energy and ambition, comes in to see me on his way to work. His girlfriend has just noticed that a large mole on his shoulder has become crusty and begun to bleed. Shortly afterwards, a young woman in a short skirt, pretty and lipsticked, comes in to tell me about the hard, irregular lump in her breast that she's just discovered in the shower that morning. She looks puzzled, but I am not. Then, later that same morning, I examine a middle-aged housewife who says that she is feeling a bit 'under the weather' – and soon my probing fingertips find the answer: an enlarged liver and spleen, and hard, swollen, rubbery glands in her groin, her neck and her armpit.

In each case I as the doctor know the plot, the likely denouement. Now my role as healer is to be a type of midwife, gently assisting in the birth of this new reality. For the patients, my presence must be constant, secure. I must never waver in my attention, even though sometimes I know that it will not help. I refer them to a hospital, and watch as they are rapidly sucked into its bottomless vortex. They tell me about all their many hospital appointments, and I receive reports from many different specialists. I talk the patients through these letters and the ambiguous words of their frowning specialists. Again I try to be constant, secure, compassionate. I try to keep my own despair at bay. I reassure them about the multiple blood tests, scans and biopsies that they will still have to endure. Often I watch, over the months, as they are weakened by chemotherapy, radiotherapy or surgery. Again I reassure them, quoting statistics and other facts, some irrelevant but others not. I try to be constant, secure, to treat their physical symptoms – but always, always, to listen to their fears and their anger.

If it turns out badly, I try to remember – as they become thinner and balder, and turn into Belsen people – what they once looked like, the first day I ever saw them. And to speak to that person, to the archaeological remains of that healthy person, as well as to their withered double lying in the bed before me. Often I am able to give them good news. My relief is great. I crack a joke. The despair lifts, at least for a while. The streets outside the Medical Centre seem suddenly suffused with light.

But at other time, I find myself sitting at a silent bedside while clocks tick rapidly away in the background, and I want to scream or to cry. But of course I say nothing. I remain constant. I only say:

'You're looking much stronger today. That's good! I'll pop in to see you again tomorrow. Or earlier, if you need me.'

I go out of the room. I take a deep breath. I drive slowly away.

Driving home, I often think about Samuel Johnson's stern warning to doctors, two centuries ago, and wonder whether he was right or not. 'I deny the lawfulness of telling a lie to a sick man for fear of alarming him,' wrote Johnson. 'You have no business with consequences; you are to tell the truth. Besides you may not be sure what effect your telling him that he is in danger may have. It may bring his distemper to a crisis, and that may cure him. Of all lying I have the greatest abhorrence of this, because I believe it has been frequently practised on myself.'

It sounds OK as a general rule but sometimes, and quite often, I find myself strongly disagreeing with him. I disagree with him because

I know, from long and bitter experience, that some patients can be killed by an overdose of truth – possibly most of them.

But then, on the other hand, there are times when I find myself agreeing with him after all. There's just no simple answer. It all depends.

Sometimes the battle to keep your patients on this side of the membrane is not just a battle with disease, but also one with the language attached to that disease. For many diseases are also metaphors: diseases of words as well as of flesh, metaphors that can wound or weaken the patient or sometimes even kill them, words that can make them lose all hope of any recovery, or else isolate them from other people, causing them to be shunned and avoided. Trapped inside a metaphor, patients can find themselves being forced to stand for something else, besides themselves. Cancer can be an example of this. So is AIDS.

In *Illness as Metaphor*, Susan Sontag has written how metaphors tend to attach mostly to serious diseases, where both their cause and outcome are unclear. In the 19th century, for example, syphilis, tuberculosis and cancer were all often used as metaphors for individual evil, while 'plague' in the popular mind was a symbol for chaos and for the breakdown of ordered society. Tuberculosis, or 'consumption' – seen then as a state of low energy and excessive sensitivity (many 19th century poets had the disease) – was often contrasted with cancer, a condition of excessive, unrestrained energy: a primitive, demonic, 'malignant' force that could somehow break down and destroy both individuals and society.

Even today, the anthropologist Deborah Gordon has described in her research in Italy how many women with breast cancer still describe it in demonic terms: as a 'plague', an epidemic, a malevolent force that has somehow invaded them from outside. It's 'a thing in the air', they say, 'a monster', 'a beast', 'an animal' that has entered their bodies without any cause and is now devouring and destroying them. This attitude often matches the use of the word 'cancer' in the media and in popular discourse, as a metaphor for spreading crime, terrorism, social breakdown or immoral behaviour. Such demonic metaphors are dangerous. They add layers of fear, to an already fearful situation. And they demand from the doctor a new approach – to treat unruly language as vigorously as you would treat unruly cells.

Sometimes, after a patient has finally crossed the membrane, I find that their medical notes seemed to have subtly changed. That they feel lifeless and limp in my hands. The ink on the tan-coloured folder seems to have faded a little, the pages have become as flimsy as onion skin. Even their surface now feels colder to the touch and drier. It's like the story by Katherine Mansfield, *Daughters of the Late Colonel*, where the photographs of the dead fade soon after their death. First the person dies, she writes, then their photograph.

Of course, it's all an illusion. But still, there is something quite unsettling about handling those records, paper echoes of patients who can never be cured, detailed narratives of a life but without any living person attached. I often find myself thinking that they need to be decently interred somewhere, just like their owners – in the capacious records department of the National Health Service, for example. And soon they are.

We all need membranes, symbolic boundaries between realities, especially between this world and the next. Sometimes the doctor's job is to provide the final seal on those boundaries, to give closure to the event, often physically as well as psychologically.

One day I am called to the house of an old woman who has just died. The family are gathered around her. It is the end of a long life and everyone has been expecting it. The old woman is lying peacefully in her bed, her eyes wide open, staring sightlessly at the ceiling. I put down my medical bag and examine her. She is still warm. But there are no movements, no breath sounds or heartbeats to be heard, no response to pain, and the pupils are fixed and dilated. She has crossed the final membrane and will never return again. I straighten up, shake my head, and mutter a few standard words of condolence. Then I pick up my bag and begin to walk towards the door, but my way is blocked. For the family have placed themselves firmly between me and the door – a solid phalanx of weeping daughters and granddaughters, of sombre sons and sons-in-law – crowded at the doorway, preventing me from leaving. I can feel them all staring at me. What do they want? What are they waiting for? What do they want me to do? There's nothing in the medical textbooks about this. No one has ever told me what to do in such a situation. We stand in a silent *tableau vivant*. It is an impasse. Minutes seem to pass, even hours. They are still waiting for me to do something, but *what*?

Suddenly Hollywood comes to my rescue. I remember all those movies I have seen, and all those final Death Scenes, the ones where comrades or friends gather round the victim at the very last moment. Then there's the dying person's final, mumbled speech in close-up, filling the screen, a few last words, a confession, a secret, the solution to a mystery, maybe a wish. And then, usually midway through a sentence, the head lolling suddenly to one side, eyes staring straight ahead, as though someone had suddenly switched off the current or pulled out the plug. But then someone else moves quickly forward into the frame, someone who walks up to the dead person with two fingers outstretched, and then gently, delicately, they…

I look around me. I am still standing in the middle of the room, and the old woman is still lying on the bed, staring upwards. And they still won't let me leave. I turn, put down my bag and slowly, gently – very delicately – pull her eyelids downwards with my two fingers until they are closed. Suddenly, the tension in the room disappears. Everyone relaxes. The tableau breaks into life and movement. People thank me tearfully, others shake my hand, some slap me on the back. Carrying my bag, I walk quickly through them, as they part like the waves of the Red Sea. Down the stairs I quickly go, then out to my car. Mission accomplished. I never, ever thought I would say it. I'm almost ashamed to say it, but now I do: 'Thank you Hollywood'.

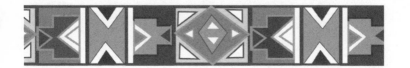

PART
3

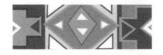

States of the Art

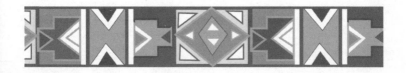

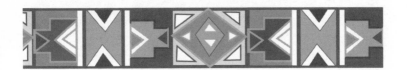

CHAPTER
17

Grand Rounds

It's one of the great rituals of modern medical life, and I am part of it. Looking around me, I can see that almost all the Consultants are men. They are specialists on every part of the body: the heart, the head, the liver, the womb. They wear dark suits and shiny black shoes, and several of them are wearing bow-ties. Among them are a few women, in smart charcoal trouser suits and fluffy white blouses, most with tiny earrings and minimal make-up. Every Monday afternoon, they all occupy the first three rows of the big lecture hall in the local hospital, for the weekly Grand Rounds, the academic centre of the week.

Behind the Consultants sit the local general practitioners (one of whom is me) – two rows of tired-looking men and women. We are wearing rougher clothes – tweeds and brogues or other sensible shoes. Unlike the Consultants, our clothing styles are more individual, but the colours are also more muted: country greys and greens and browns, sometimes black or dark blue. Bleepers rest in our pockets or handbags, chirping occasionally like agitated birds. Medical bags rest on our laps or under our seats. All of us family doctors are tired, but alert. Most of us are on call.

Behind us, the rest of the hall is a mass of white coats and name-tags. First come the Senior Registrars or Residents, the rising stars, hungry for attention and for promotion. Then the Junior Registrars and the Senior House Officers, and then behind them all the mass of interns or House Officers, with their crumpled white coats and exhausted faces, their bleepers going off every few moments, coat pockets stuffed with textbooks, stethoscopes and patella hammers. And finally behind them, crowded uncomfortably into an invisible ghetto in the last few rows of the hall, and sitting silently in their white coats without name-tags, are all the foreign medical graduates. They are at the very bottom of the food chain, and they know it. They are attached to this hospital only for extra postgraduate courses, while they study for their British medical exams. They form a group of generally older men and women, who talk quietly among themselves in Urdu or Arabic, Farsi or Gujurati. Scattered around the hall, too, are a few medical students, sitting awkwardly in their half-length white coats, conscious of the fact that they are only half a doctor, and therefore entitled to only half a coat.

The lecture hall is a miniature of the English class system, or at least of the class system that existed at the time of the British Empire. In the outside world, all that has largely disappeared. But for some reason it still survives here, embalmed within the disinfected walls of this small suburban hospital.

One after another, the nurses bring in the Interesting Cases, pushing them in wheelchairs onto the little stage in front, or guiding them gently forward, together with the stand of intravenous fluid that accompanies them. Others appear in their hospital beds, wheeled in by two or three sweating porters. One by one they are announced by the Consultant whose day it is. Today it's all about gastroenterology, and the big florid man in the crimson bow-tie is centre stage. He has lots of juicy cases to show us: ulcerative colitis, intestinal obstruction, an odd case of gallstones, a burst peptic ulcer, a stomach cancer that is spreading much too fast and unexpectedly soon.

The Consultant briefly introduces each Interesting Case to the assembled crowd. He tells them about the puzzle of diagnosis they represent, the difficulties of treatment he and his team have encountered. He poses one diagnostic puzzle, and then another. Each case is a complex riddle, one that only he can solve. But not quite yet. For first he must show us all the dimensions of the mystery: the ambiguous blood tests, the misleading ultra-sound scans, the confusing X-ray findings, the clinical signs that (of course) 'the GP' missed and the junior doctors never spotted – until, that is, he took a better look. It is not surprising that Arthur Conan Doyle was a doctor, for each case is presented here as a Sherlock Holmes mystery. There's that sudden, unexpected call on the Consultant's services. They need his help, urgently. He reluctantly agrees to take on the case. The GP in this story plays the bumbling Inspector Lestrade, the baffled junior hospital doctor is Dr Watson, while he – of course – is... Adjusting his deer-stalker hat and pipe, he asks the patient a pointed question or two, but expects only a very short answer in reply.

'Tell the doctors, Mr Biggs, when exactly it was that you noticed the change in your bowel movements. Don't be nervous now, they want to know.'

Sometimes, speaking quickly, he adds, 'Any questions, anyone?', but allows only one or two brief queries, before signalling to the nurses to wheel Mr Biggs away. Occasionally, one of the Interesting Patients breaks the script, talks too much, reveals too much or even cracks a joke. Then the Consultant becomes tense, his face serious and stern. He signals frantically to the nurses. He thanks the patient effusively for coming to talk to them. And then makes sure that they wheel him quickly away.

After the patients leave, a detailed discussion of the cases takes place, almost entirely among the Consultants. They talk only among themselves, hardly glancing behind them at the rest of the packed hall, their voices often inaudible to the rest of us. Occasionally a bright young Senior Registrar – a rising star and Consultant-in-waiting – rises to ask a question, a searching, clever, informed question, laced with impressive quotations from the latest editions of *The Lancet*, the *British Medical Journal* or *Advances in Gastroenterology*. The Consultants listen respectfully, a tolerant – but uneasy – smile on their faces. And soon Grand Rounds is over.

Grand Rounds can be enjoyed as theatre, a weekly mystery play. Some of the Consultants – clever storytellers that they are – hide the solution, the true diagnosis, right to very end. With them on the podium, you can almost hear those gasps of surprise and pleasure, at the eventual arrival of the denouement ('Good Lord, so it *was* myelofibrosis after all, not aplastic anaemia!'). If the Consultant is skilful enough, he will maintain the tension almost to the last moment, before dissolving it with his brilliant solution, plucking it out of his top hat, as it were, and then taking a bow: 'Elementary, my dear Watson!'

Grand Rounds also has another, more hidden function – as important for the participants as the sharing of medical knowledge. They can also be seen as a ritual of healing for the doctors themselves, a way of dealing with ambiguity and doubt, and with the daily traumas of disease and death in medical practice. Each week the Grand Rounds, with their standardised genre of stories – each beginning with mystery and doubt but almost all ending in diagnostic certainty – impose some sense of order, of a coherent narrative, onto the unpredictability of human suffering that the doctors encounter. It's a great way of reducing anxiety, of reducing uncertainty to the certainty of numbers. For people whose professional lives are spent among so much suffering, pain, trauma and ambiguity, Grand Rounds poses cosmic riddles, but it also solves them. It gives meaning and coherence to what has happened, reassuring the audience that, seen through the lens of medicine, the world does after all make sense. And if, at the end of the afternoon, the meaning of life is still not clear, then at least they can give you the precise cause of death. For in the medical world-view everything does have a cause – a *why* – even if that cause is for the moment idiopathic, unknown.

I usually enjoy these weekly presentations. I actually like the 'hard science' of medicine that they reveal, and not just the touchy-feely aspects. All those charts and diagrams and statistics, and fascinating glimpses of the body's inner secrets – it's a finite, explicable world up there, projected onto the screen. In the face of suffering, science is a comforting world-view.

But in this particular hospital, the weekly display of medical hierarchy often goes together with a certain ritual, but polite, humiliation of 'the GP'. This mythological figure appears as a minor character in several of the case presentations: as a figure of fun, the Joker in the pack, the bumbling, well-meaning generalist with suppos-edly limited diagnostic skills ('The GP, of course, thought it was only a cold', 'I'm afraid the GP just gave him some cough medicine, and sent him home,' 'The GP only referred him to us, when it was already much too late'). Many of the Consultants in this hall seem to see the local GPs as honest craftsmen and artisans: decent, well-meaning folk, but not 'real' gentlemen – or 'real' medical scientists – like themselves.

In Britain, all these peculiar prejudices have a long history. Back in the Middle Ages the precursors of today's general practitioners were specialised tradesmen called apothecaries. From 1617 onwards they were licensed to sell drugs prescribed by the physicians, though only in 1703 were they entitled to see patients themselves and to prescribe for them directly. From then on they became the GPs of the poorer classes. Right from the early days, the physicians saw themselves as the only 'real' doctors around, superior both to these apothecaries and to the surgeons, those mere 'sawbones', with their long knives and scalpels and blood-stained coats. The growth of the big public hospitals from about 1700 onwards enhanced the position of both physicians and surgeons, but not that of the apothecaries or their present-day descendants, the general practitioners or family doctors.

Still, unlike US doctors, British family doctors in the last century or so have retained an important share of primary care (especially after the National Insurance Act of 1911 and the establishment of the National Health Service in 1948). Even today, about 60 per cent of doctors in the UK are general practitioners. Meanwhile, on the other side of the Atlantic, the 'old-time family doctor' portrayed in the famous painting by Norman Rockwell, has all but disappeared.

Even among the so-called 'real doctors', the Consultants, there is a strict hierarchy, based on the conditions they treat and the parts of the body they focus on. Among surgeons for example, the symbolic value we in the Western world give to those two key organs – the brain and the heart – puts brain surgeons and heart surgeons much higher in the professional pecking order than rectal surgeons, urologists, gynaecologists or the rest.

The year I spend as a Visiting Fellow at Harvard Medical School illuminates some of the social differences between Britain and the USA – and their two medical systems. My first Grand Rounds at one of the Harvard teaching hospitals takes place only a few days after my wife and I arrive in August in hot, humid Boston.

It's lunchtime, and the auditorium is packed. A bespectacled sea of white coats, beepers and name-tags: attending physicians, interns, residents and a few nurses. Scattered among them are several family doctors, but like the specialists they too are wearing white coats. And then there are the medical students, awkward in their familiar half-coats.

Today, too, it's the turn of gastroenterology. And the attending physician in that specialty takes the podium. As with his British counterpart, it's his special time now and he intends to make the very most of it. Under his white coat he wears a plaid shirt and a red tie. He is clever and witty and bald, wears thick horn-rimmed glasses and tells risqué jokes. It appears that he, too, has read Arthur Conan Doyle.

Today he is discussing a particular case, an especially taxing diagnostic mystery – something in the stomach or in the oesophagus. He gives a brief history of the patient, his puzzling presentation, the unusual configuration of his symptoms. Then onto the screen he projects one slide after another – of the patient's X-rays, ultra-sound scans and barium meals, his blood tests and bacteriological swabs. As they flash up there, in technicolour profusion, the mystery deepens. You can feel the tension rising. Everyone laughs even louder at his jokes; their attention is undivided. Then he shows a video of his endoscopic examination of the patient. Up on the screen we watch as the camera on its long fibre-optic stalk tunnels down the moist, heaving pink interior of the patient's oesophagus (reminding me of Don Marquis's famous quip: 'Time the anthropophagous, swallows down all human works through his broad esophagus!') – then down into his stomach and his duodenum. Thanks to diagnostic technology, it's an Incredible Voyage of discovery into the pink, mysterious interior of a living human being.

To my surprise, during the discussion of the cases several junior doctors – even interns – raise issues and ask searching questions. They don't seem embarrassed to do so. The grey-haired Chiefs of Department and attending physicians are in charge, of course, but the medical hierarchy here seems to be much less rigid than in England. Or else it is better disguised. But I find myself feeling more and more uncomfortable. Where is that human being? When will they bring him in? Where is the patient?

I look around me, but there is no one to be seen. I look at my watch.

The Grand Rounds are almost over. Everyone is still transfixed by the screen. I lean over to one of the attending physicians sitting beside me.

'But where's the patient?' I ask, 'When are they going to bring him in?'

The man looks at me askew. My accent, my lack of a white coat, my question puzzle him.

'The patient?' he asks, frowning, shaking his head in disbelief, 'The *patient?!*'

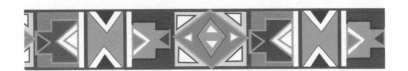

CHAPTER
18

Healing Time

Each time I return to Cape Town, I re-visit the South African Museum in the old Botanical Gardens, near the centre of town. It's my favourite place. On the left as you enter is the large hall of Bushmen rock paintings, close to the dinosaur room. Great slabs of flat rock, cut from the walls of remote mountain caves and crevices, are mounted behind glass. Bright, beautiful panoramas – each one an African Lascaux – they are the ancient cave paintings of the San people, the earliest inhabitants of southern Africa. Across these irregular rocky landscapes you can make out groups of tiny stick-like figures, hunters and gatherers, men and women – stalking or striding among herds of eland and kudu, past leopards, giraffes, elephants and antelope. In one of the larger paintings, a shaman lies prone on the ground, deep in a trance, his head surrounded by a corona of fish and eels. Fish and eels – in the middle of the veldt? But for the San this image apparently had a very specific meaning, for they saw trance as a state similar to being underwater, with every perception shifting and blurred. They also believed, apparently, that the painted rock itself was only the outer surface of the events it portrayed, and that these events continued into the spirit world, deep inside it.

Recently, I saw a book of exact reproductions of these cave paintings. Each had been painted *in situ* using ochre, ash and other natural pigments. Paging through these exquisite images, I realise why they provoke in me not only admiration, but also a certain unease. For in the darkness of the deepest caves or overhangs, most of the painting would have been hidden in shadow. Neither the San nor their shaman would ever see all of the painting at the same time. Only the slow movement of the sun as it migrated across the enormous sky would reveal it, inch by inch. Beginning in the cool dewy, chirping morning, through the suffocating heat of the African noon and the lengthening shadows of late afternoon, the sun would touch on one part of the irregular surface after another. Depending on when you looked, you could usually see only one episode of the total story at a time. In this, as in similar art books, the experience of cave art has been irreversibly changed. Time, space, and the cycles of the day and the year, have all been flattened out. They have been condensed by our modern, impatient gaze into an eternal present. Everything is synchronic, immediate. The experience now is clear, flat and simultaneous.

It may seem fanciful, but this image of the sun moving slowly across the cave painting, revealing one bit after another, somehow reminds me of the differences between two types of medical care: family practice and hospital medicine. On the one hand is family medicine with its slow revelation to the doctor of a life pattern, or a pattern of disease, in an individual or a family. On the other is the image of a person revealed instantaneously in a hospital clinic by the technology of scientific medicine: X-rays, scans, MRIs, blood tests – and often in a rushed consultation between two strangers. It's the fundamental difference between the briefest glimpse and a lengthy narrative. Between a snapshot and a long novel. As with the Bushman paintings, it means translating the irregular, evolving texture of a life into the synchronic flatness of a piece of paper.

Today, this snapshot medicine is winning the battle, not old-style general practice. And I deeply regret this. For medicine lives increasingly in a synchronic age, an age of immediacy. Time is different now, and patients have become '*im*patients', expecting quick fixes and instant cures. The symptom of the moment is everything, future and past are largely irrelevant. Time is *now*.

I think of these changes as symbolised not only by that book on Bushman art, but also by the common wristwatch and the way that this small, familiar, circular object – with its mildly anthropomorphic 'face', its minute and second 'hands' – has now become transformed into the digital watch. And how this in turn parallels a shift from the traditional idea of time as circular (and repetitive) to the absolute immediacy of numbers. From a glimpse of past, present and future – time before the present moment, and time still to come – to the instantaneous moment, the *now*.

It's the same with our current obsession with genetics. Genes in the present encapsulate the past as well as the future. At any moment they contain within them not only all the legacy of inherited disorders and genetic tendencies, but also the potential for future diseases. Like the digital watch, the information they store at any one moment compresses past and future, into the eternal present.

In contrast to all this, old-style family medicine (like traditional medicine) has always worked with a much longer and evolving sense of time. In their medical centres and offices and surgeries, family doctors see, sitting across the desk from them, all the cycles of life unfolding – children growing up, parents getting older, birth, adolescence, marriage and death, whether fast or slow, anticipated or not. They watch the sweet babies they once immunised against measles and diphtheria metamorphosing into moody and pimply teenagers, and then gradually into the surly parents of a new generation of sweet-faced babies. Family medicine moves effortlessly from nappy rashes and feeding problems to pre-school vaccinations, from sniffles and coughs up to period problems and adolescent acne; from the first tentative talk about contraception (perhaps even the morning-after-pill) to creams and lotions to clear the skin before the Big Date, that important dance, or even the Big Wedding. Every day it moves across the generations, as the cycle of life turns on itself, and then begins all over again. Along the way it offers the family doctor a series of brief glimpses of each patient, sometimes (at least in the National Health system) only a few minutes long, spread over very many years. But spliced together, fed into a projector and then speeded up, the narrative of a life emerges clearly on the screen – a little jerky and scratched in places, but a true human story nevertheless.

Some of these life stories of patients make sense only over a much longer period, years perhaps or even generations. Using a genogram, a sort of family tree of symptoms, you can show how symptoms percolate down through an individual's life, and also through a particular family history, picked up like the baton in a relay race in each generation, and then handed on – especially stress or psychosomatic symptoms. Often a genogram can reveal a genealogy of 'tension headaches', 'nervous stomachs' or 'irritable bowels' that stretch over several generations. Similarly it can chart a 'headache family', or one specialising in 'digestive problems' (often one whose emotional dramas always take place at mealtimes), or a family where the solution to every problem always comes out of a bottle or a syringe. You can track inherited habits of drug use, divorce, domestic violence, alcoholism or teenage pregnancy – and the tragic spoor that they leave behind. You can see clearly how some families mature over time like a good wine, while others turn slowly into vinegar.

Often you find that it is *time* that is the true healer of a body, or of a family, and not any medical 'quick fix' – time as a force of Nature, advancing or retreating, healing some people, destroying others – so that the wise doctor learns eventually to work in alliance with it. In many cases, as the sardonic Voltaire once remarked: 'The art of medicine consists in amusing the patient while nature cures the disease.'

Family medicine also teaches another truth: that many patients are bilingual. For when you get to know them well, over many years, you realise that over time people and their bodies can speak in two distinct languages, and that they often say very different things. Eventually you learn to pick up these dissonant messages, even though sometimes it's like a film in which the dialogue, and the subtitles printed below it, don't quite agree with one another.

The alcoholic angrily denies that he's still drinking. His face is flushed and emphatic. He says he is hurt by your lack of trust in him. Don't you believe him? But when his body is allowed to 'speak' directly to the doctor through a blood test, it tells a very different story – especially his liver. Its voice on the liver function tests is often shrill and desperate. It's hurt, damaged, becoming cirrhotic with despair. Its voice, amplified by the lab tests, sings a very different song from that of its owner.

Another patient, apparently healthy, suddenly gets gravely ill. And when you hear this, you're surprised that you're really not surprised. Somehow you always 'knew' that this would happen, that they would develop cancer, or heart disease, or have a stroke, or whatever. Somehow you just knew, even though there was no scientific evidence, no possible 'risk factors'. And yet on some subliminal level you heard the low, whispered voice of their disease speaking to you, long, long before it showed up in their tests.

Mrs D is a mysterious woman. I have known her for many years, yet never been able to puzzle her out. Each time I see her, I feel uneasy afterwards. But why? She is elderly and frail, her speech is quiet and flat and sometimes difficult to follow. She rarely smiles; she doesn't respond to small talk; she rarely even makes eye contact. She's there in my room, and yet she's not there. And yet she's not clinically depressed – the psychiatrists assure me of that. But she always seems to be elsewhere, a woman living in another story, another drama, but not in this particular story here, the one taking place now in my consulting room. Every time I ask her if there's something wrong in her life, she denies it firmly.

'There's nothing wrong in my life,' she says. 'Everything is really fine. No problems. Everything at home is going OK. '

She comes in frequently to see me with this symptom or with that. Dozens of them. Almost all of them have no physical basis, and the examination and laboratory tests are always negative. And yet, and yet... The feeling that I am missing something, that something is being 'said' to me in a subliminal way, gets stronger each time I see her, each time she presents herself with yet another inexplicable symptom. Is it just simple hypochondria, or is something else going on?

Years go by. On the surface, nothing changes. And yet one day it all *does* comes out. Without warning, she opens up to me. For the first time, I understand the story that she has been living in, the message that her body was trying to tell me. It's a distant story, in a far-away land, and she's lived within it secretly for many decades now. To some extent, she still is living there.

It appears that during the Second World War she was living in a city in South-East Asia, where she and her husband ran a small family business. They had one son, about 13. Then one day the Japanese invaded. Thousand of troops in khaki uniforms fought their way into the city outskirts, Zero fighters screamed overhead. There was panic and confusion. People ran screaming here and there. The air was filled with black smoke, dead bodies lay strewn in the streets. She and her husband were trapped by the attack at their business, in the centre of town. They had left their son at home that day, together with the servant. By the time they managed to return to the house, through the burning vehicles and the shattered glass, it was empty. Her son and the servant were gone. They searched and searched, but soon she and her husband were forced to flee to save their lives, to join the crowds of other refugees streaming out of the city. She never saw him again. After the War, she returned to the city, and began searching for her son again. She had posters with his photograph on printed, and then pasted up on walls, temples and trees, all over that part of South-East Asia. For years the search went on. But there were never any leads. Her son was never found.

Eventually they moved to London, where she had a few relatives. For years she has carried the photograph of the smiling 13-year old boy pasted inside herself. For years she has carried on the search. The child within her never ages, but always smiles back at her from the poster. Sometimes the pain of that smile is almost too much to bear. She never discusses it, or him, with anyone else. Hardly anyone, except for her husband, knows what she is carrying around within her. And despite knowing her all those years, until that moment, I never knew. Only now, after many years, does she feel safe enough to reveal her secret pain. Now she seems relieved, relaxed. She even, for the first time, smiles a little at me. We both feel a deep relaxation between us. We talk freely together, for the first time, and for a long time. Not for the first time do I realise that, in family medicine, time can be the best form of diagnosis, even of treatment.

Mrs D shows me how people can hold within themselves the dead voices of their past. When I think of her, I think also of Natalie Cole, singing a duet with the recorded voice of her dead father, Nat King Cole, many years after his death. *Unforgettable* is a moving song, one that compresses time, denying the everlasting silence of death. Like the digital watch, it's the past and present, fused into one.

That song, like family medicine itself, has taught me that each human body is a palimpsest, one into which many different voices and stories and scripts have been inscribed. Often you can track these stories as they move slowly through a person's biography, like wind through a cornfield, moving through patterns of work and love and leisure, penetrating every aspect of their life, and then in some cases settling eventually, like a toxic cloud, into their cells, hormones or coronary arteries – or into their psyches.

When Sally reaches 55, the same age at which her mother had died of a heart attack, she becomes unaccountably depressed. Her life is OK, but now she worries all the time, especially about her heart. She imagines pains, pressures, palpitations, spasms, tightness and other uncomfortable feelings within her chest. Her breath becomes short, she pants with the slightest exertion. Sally knows for sure that soon she is going to die from a heart attack, just as her mother did. She can hear that message of doom inscribed clearly in the walls of her coronary arteries and in the frantic beat and flow of her blood. Four times that year she goes to see a cardiologist. Each time many blood tests and cardiograms are done, angiograms too. But nothing is ever found. Her heart is fine they say. After each set of tests, her symptoms improve for a while, only to recur with redoubled force. But at the end of that 55th year, all her symptoms disappear. She's still alive. The curse has expired.

Sally gives a great sigh of relief, as the sun moves on and that big herd of kudus – with their long, pointed, dangerous horns – move slowly out of sight, and then into the shadows.

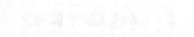

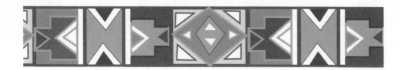

CHAPTER
19

Hospital

It's a cool autumn evening. After giving a lecture to anthropology students at Cambridge University about cultural perceptions of the body, I return home yawning and exhausted, trip down the stairs, and smash my ankle. It's a bad break, a bi-malleolar fracture, and when I look down at it, the ankle is flapping helplessly to and fro. One side of it bulges and sags strangely, as though it were made of wax and has been left out to melt in the summer sun. I watch curiously as it slowly turns purplish-blue and yellowish, speckled all over with red blotches like an *avant garde* painting. Later in hospital, when they show me the X-ray of my ankle, all the dispersed and irregular fragments of white bone floating against a dark background remind me only of one thing: an aerial view of the Greek Islands.

The ambulance-men wheel me into the Accident and Emergency Department on a trolley. The corridors are grey, the floors a shiny blue linoleum, the air cool and filled with unfamiliar smells. Signs whiz past, pointing to 'Radiology', 'Medical Imaging', 'Fracture Clinic'. There is noise and shouting, the clink of instruments, and the sonorous moans of someone inside a curtained cubicle. People in white coats and green smocks rush past me, then rush back again. Somewhere there is the beep-beep-beep of monitor machines. High above my head, the clean white ceilings flow swiftly past. They have a regular grid pattern, a pattern of rectangular tiles and air vents and square fluorescent light panels. It's an ordered, precise and rational world up there, in counterpoint to all the chaos and confusion below.

More people come and go. Someone removes my jacket, someone else cuts through the leg of my trousers. A third person in a white smock, who doesn't introduce himself, gives me an injection. There are more X-rays, blood tests, forms to be signed, and an operation is arranged for the following morning. I am left lying on the trolley, waiting for a bed in the orthopaedic ward. I find myself a member of a new community. We are the Trolley People, the horizontal citizens of our own tiny world. Lying shivering under our thin blankets, we have become like a new species of centaur: half human, half trolley.

There are five or six of us, lying near to each other. We moan, we thrash about, we call out plaintively to the nurses and doctors hurrying past, but without hope that they will ever respond. We ask each other what went wrong ('So what happened to you, then?'), but never listen to the reply. We are each encapsulated within our own suffering. Sometimes we exchange tiny bits of local gossip ('Someone said there's been a big traffic accident – that's why they're all so busy tonight.'), or give helpful tips ('They say that nurse over there is nice; she can get you the newspaper, if you give her the money').

I see them with my double vision, my diplopia. They are my community now, but they are also that other, alien species: *patients*. The elderly woman over there, for example, probably has a broken femur. The young man sweating restlessly on his trolley is obviously in drug withdrawal. Someone else beside him in a torn bathrobe, naked underneath, writhes around, holding his stomach: it could be intestinal obstruction. There's a teenager, with a broken left ankle, probably just like mine; an elderly man with an intravenous drip, half comatose, waiting to be taken up to the wards – probably a stroke. All my fellow citizens. One by one they are wheeled away as the evening goes on, and others take their place. And each time we, the Trolley People, re-form into a new little community with our new members. And us Old Timers welcome these newcomers as they join us, with nods and painful smiles.

The atmosphere around us is tense, wary. Burly uniformed security men patrol the corridors. Just above my trolley a laminated notice has been tacked to the wall: 'VIOLENCE IN OUR HOSPITAL – The Hospital believes that violence, physical aggression and verbal abuse are unacceptable. If this happens against our staff or others, appropriate action – including legal action – will be taken.'

I try to imagine some violent patient on a late Friday night, crazed by too many drugs – or too few – pausing to read it through, reading the words carefully through his contracted pupils, then taking a deep breath and quickly returning to his seat, now docile and calm.

Eventually they wheel me off to the X-ray Department and leave me there in a deserted corridor. Suddenly blood begins to gush and pump out of the cannula they have inserted into my arm. It spreads quickly across the blanket, the trolley and much of my shirt. But there is no one to call for help. I am quite alone. I watch the blood spreading. It looks cinematic, unreal, a can of spilt paint. I call out to a passing patient. She stares wide-eyed at the spreading stain, then limps quickly out of the corridor. A few moments later, a nurse appears.

When they wheel me back to re-join the Trolley People, I feel quite proud. For a moment I hide my hospital ID card under the blanket, the one I'd been gripping as a talisman against medical indifference. My shirt is soaked now with the blood of membership, a broken, wounded member of the Casualty Club.

The Last Supper before the operation is a plate of tinned soup, a stale sandwich and a tiny tub of over-sweetened yoghurt. The next morning I wake up, my head throbbing, toxic with chemicals: pre-med, anaesthetic gases, morphine and a heavy injection of antibiotics. Also self-blame, anxiety and guilt. My ankle, the guilty one who has let me down, lies locked away in its plaster-of-paris cell, throbbing with remorse. The pain is intense with even the slightest movement, but somehow it is also curiously silent. The pain needs a voice, but not my own.

I open my eyes again.

'Good morning. How intense is your pain?' asks the young man in the white uniform, carrying a clipboard, 'Say how much out of ten would you give it?

Who is he? A nurse, I think. A pain specialist.

Twenty? Thirty? No, can't say that, he'll think I'm mad. Ten-out-often. Can't say that either; he'd think I was a neurotic, a weakling.

'Seven out of ten.'

'Oh, good. Seven, you say?'

The next day, the same question:

'How much out of ten would you give your pain?'

'Six'

'Oh, six. Good. We're making progress.'

The next day 'five'. He looks satisfied, but I am not. Shouldn't he perhaps have asked me: How are you? How are you *feeling*?

Like Kafka's Gregor Samsa, I have woken up to find myself metamorphosed. Not into a giant insect this time, but into a number – or rather, into a collage of numbers. My case number, my temperature, my height and weight, my pulse rate and blood pressure, my blood count – and the level of my pain. All of this just duplicates what is happening in the world outside. For there, too, I seem to exist increasingly as a collection of numbers: bank account, credit card, telephone, drivers licence, passport, area code, and the unique configuration of my genetic code.

Hospitals are special places. They have their own, unique gravitational fields. Caught within them, you soon find yourself as if in a science fiction film or in a dream, where the dimensions of time and space are fundamentally different. Where Space seems to distend and Time too, where everything seems further away from you than it ever was. To reach out and grab it now, seems almost impossible. Beginning at the edge of your bed, space seems to extend into infinity. And everything is not only far away, but getting further every moment, for the universe around you is expanding in all directions, but at an unknown rate. Time, too, seems to change in similar ways, especially your personal body time, the timing of needs and the satisfaction of those needs: for food, water, pain relief or the urine bottle. Some events now take place in slower motion, others too quickly to understand.

After the operation, I can't pass urine. I simply can't, even though I strain and strain. I'm a doctor, so I know what's happening. It's postoperative urinary retention, due to the anaesthetic drugs. And I also know that if it doesn't clear on its own, then I'll need to be catheterised. I try and try, my stomach beginning to swell. I can feel the upper border of the bladder rising up towards my navel, like a pregnant uterus. I call again. Nurses come and go, flustered, confused. Someone runs some water for a few minutes, on the other side of the ward, hoping that it'll stimulate a release, but it doesn't work.

I call again. No one comes. My bladder rises even further. Will it burst? The senior nurse refuses to catheterise me. She says she cannot do so without the presence of a doctor. And they're all too busy at the moment. 'Sorry', she says. They promise me they'll come in 'five minutes', then 'fifteen minutes', then 'soon'. The pain increases. My bladder rises further. I look at my watch. I've not passed water for almost six hours now. I get angry. I have to change roles. I have to stop being a patient and become a doctor again, my own doctor, otherwise I'm in danger. Eventually they call a young woman, a registrar – flustered, attractive. The nurse catheterises me: 1250 ccs of fluid burst out of me. A litre and a quarter!

The next day, I am feeling thirsty.

'I'm thirsty, really thirsty,' I say to a nurse.

'I'll get you a glass of water', she says.

But she forgets. Almost an hour passes. I am still thirsty. No one responds to my bell or my calls. No one can see me, because when she left my bed, for some reason she drew the curtains tightly closed behind her. Eventually, someone else hears my cry, brings me a big bottle of water, and then leaves, again drawing the curtains behind her. It's as if drinking water were such an intimate, shameful act, that no one else in the ward should witness it. But in my weakened state, the bottle is too heavy for me to lift up. I can't pour it into a glass without most either spilling onto the floor or onto my blankets. I can't hold it in my left hand either, because that arm's connected to an IV drip. Now there's water, water, spilling everywhere, but still hardly a drop to drink.

Eventually someone comes, and pours the water for me. Later they bring me a urine bottle, then suddenly leave – but this time leaving the curtains half-open. I am sitting half-naked, holding a urine bottle that is already full. For almost half-an-hour I sit there, holding it carefully, afraid of spilling. No one replies to my constant ringing.

'The nurses are really run off their feet today', someone says.

In the ward, things fly apart – promises, words, especially words and the actions and objects that they refer to. Everything seems to move apart, and is no longer connected to anything else. No wonder most of the other patients have now become '*im*patients': restless, angry, dissatisfied. I realise that this is what it's like to be the new post-modernist patient, to be only a collection of different organs, each one cared for by a different specialist. I am now a Babel of parts, each one unconnected to all the others. And at the centre, nothing, only an absence.

Something is missing. But what?

Whatever it is, it's not just the usual story: under-staffing, lack of resources in the National Health Service, too many demands on the medical staff, low pay and low morale. It's all of that, of course, but also more than that. And certainly it's not just me. Over the years I've heard literally hundreds of similar stories from my patients and friends, and even written and taught about the subject, but somehow never quite believed it all. And yet one thing is for sure: in the hospital, something in us is missing. Something at the very core of us. Some essence of who we are is now absent. We have become partial people, treated only in a partial way. We are now just broken limbs, diseased organs, collections of unruly cells. We are pieces of people, fragments, shards, sharp splinters, only the sum of our parts. Something is missing. Call it 'person' or even 'spirit' or 'soul', but whatever it is you cannot see it under the microscope, or spot it on a CAT scan. You can't measure it or photograph it, and yet it's always present. We lie there in the hospital ward like a row of pale human bagels, each one of us hollow in the middle.

I recall Oliver Sacks's horrifying account, in his book *A Leg to Stand On*, of his hospitalisation for a serious leg injury, of what he describes as the 'systematic depersonalisation which goes with becoming-a-patient'. He sees all of this humiliation, this stripping away of all personal identity, dignity and control, as analogous to becoming a prisoner, or to a child's first day at school. 'And I was seized, over-whelmed, by this dread,' he writes, 'this elemental sense and dread of degradation'.

But it's not just the doctors. They are like kindly but absent fathers, who dart into the wards, examine or treat a few patients, and then disappear again, leaving the ongoing care to the nurses. But that's how they've always been. And all the orthopaedic surgeons I encounter are skilful and good at their job. They are not just the carpenters and technicians of the mass-production medical system, which is the National Health Service. Somewhat to my surprise, they take the time to explain to me exactly what has happened, and why, and what is now likely to happen. They describe the operation to come in some detail, and what has to be done to repair the ankle firmly. They use words like 'pins', 'plates' and 'screws' – familiar, domestic words, which from now on will always have a different meaning for me.

Meanwhile, in their clean starched uniforms, the nurses move quickly past my bed, harassed, angry and over-stretched. They rush and snap. Many seem to have withdrawn from their caring role, or else been forced out of it. Everyone knows they are under-paid, over-worked, under-valued. But I think of all those intimate family words we used to associate with them – 'sister', 'matron', 'nurse' – and how difficult it is to apply these words to them any more or, at least, to the ones I encounter in this particular ward and in this particular hospital. And we now need a new family vocabulary for the male nurses, the kindest of all. No, it's not really the nurses' fault either. So what is it, then?

One answer is that hospitals have become factories, yet another form of industrial mass-production in our society, with the raw material of Sick People being fed in at one end, and Healthy People being produced *en masse* at the other. Or at least, that's the aim. But they turn us from people into products at a very crucial time in our lives, a time of anxiety and ambiguity, where the very threads that hold our sense of personhood together are in danger of being torn apart. Many hospitals have become businesses, dedicated solely to production – if not to profit, to cost effectiveness – but without considering the other types of cost that result from this approach: social, emotional, spiritual. They have become businesses run by managers, primarily for the benefit of other managers, accountants and of other executives higher up in the food chain. No wonder so many patients are unhappy with hospitals these days. Nor is it surprising, as I have read that in the USA in 1960 there was one hospital administrator for every 3.17 patients, but that by 1990 this had risen to one patient for every 1.43 administrators. And in all of this, the suffering of an individual patient, with all its mess and unpredictability, can often get in the way.

A week or so later, we reassemble at the Fracture Clinic. With our crutches and plaster casts, we are a ragged crowd of three-legged animals, a herd of hopping, stumbling, slipping creatures. We, the former Trolley People, pretend now not to recognise each other. The receptionist calls my name, and I limp forward obediently. Again, a nurse leaves me lying alone in a small room and then disappears. Again she closes the door behind her. A half-hour passes. I'm feeling cold, shivery. Where is she? And where is the doctor?

Things fly apart, disintegrate. Space and Time. Events once linked together in the old world, now have drifted apart: words and actions, far from each other. I'm thinking: 'I'll go the toilet', or 'I'll get a glass of water', but then nothing happens. Nothing moves.

In this hospital, at least, it seems that no one is interested any longer in putting the shattered pieces of Humpty-Dumpty back together again.

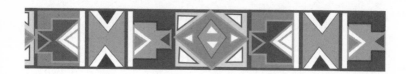

CHAPTER
20

Paradigm Lost

Standing around the bedside, they teach us carefully how actually to examine a patient. It is an important part of the training at our medical school in Cape Town, perhaps the most important part. We learn to use our senses, every one of them, not only to hear the patient's story ('the History'), but also to look carefully at their body, to touch it, to feel it here and there, to smell the breath for signs of diabetic acidosis, to listen intently to the timbre of their breathing. Gradually we learn to use our eyes, nose, ears and fingertips, as well as our memory and intuition. We strain to use every single one of these senses to make the diagnosis, to sense the secrets that lie beneath the skin.

Our tutors show us how to examine a patient's chest, in a particular and ritualised way, to memorise a type of mantra: *Inspection – Palpation – Percussion – Auscultation*. One after the other, to look at the chest, to touch it, to tap it – and only then to listen to the lungs or heart with our stethoscopes. Instruments and diagnostic machines had to come second then, not first, as they sometimes do today. But before the physical examination always comes the History, the patient's particular narrative.

I thought that it had always been so, this way of collecting information from a patient, but I was wrong. According to medical historians, it was only in the 19th century that doctors actually began to examine their patients' bodies in any detail. Before that time they would observe them closely, occasionally take their pulse or inspect their tongue, or peer at their urine or stools. But mostly they relied on the patient's account of what had happened. Eliciting this detailed 'history' of their illness, watching for inconsistencies or omissions, and trying to guess at the 'true' meaning of what was said, all made medical diagnosis into a type of literary criticism. For a long time, medicine was all about *stories*, not only the patient's 'history' and the doctor's 'diagnosis', but also the mingling of these two narratives in the medical consultation.

'There's no need for fiction in medicine,' says Dr Foster, the general practitioner in Arthur Conan Doyle's story *A Medical Document*, 'for the facts will always beat anything you can fancy.' Dr Foster was right. There is no end to the human dramas that walk through the doctor's door, the extraordinary range of personal 'histories'. And not surprisingly, many doctors themselves are natural storytellers, and many have actually become writers: from Rabelais, Celine, Somerset Maugham, William Carlos Williams, Oliver Sacks, Arthur Conan Doyle, A.J. Cronin, Richard Selzer, Robin Cook, Ethan Canin, Mikhail Bulgakov, Anton Chekhov – up to Michael Crichton, creator of *ER* and *Jurassic Park*.

Growing up as I did in a medical family, this atmosphere of medical tale-telling was familiar to me. As a child I would watch as clinical stories and 'case-histories' bounced round the room, one after another, each beginning just as another one ended. 'That's the worst of these medical stories,' complains the outsider in Conan Doyle's story, listening in, 'they never seem to have an end.'

But even among doctors, some medical stories seem to form a special genre of their own. These are tales about their most difficult patients, the ones with bizarre complaints or impossible symptoms. Like the denizens of some medieval bestiary, these eccentric or hypochondriacal patients – often called 'Fat File' or 'Heart-Sink' patients – are wondered at, compared and minutely discussed, often with the tiniest shudder.

In 1922 my uncle Louis Mirvish, later an eminent gastroenterologist, was one of the first two doctors to graduate in South Africa. (Before then, you could only begin your medical training there, before completing it in Britain, Germany or the Netherlands). When Uncle Louis first entered the University of Cape Town Medical School in 1917, the practice of medicine was very different to what it is today. The X-ray had been discovered by Röntgen only twenty years or so before, and there were no endoscopies then, and no CAT scans or MRIs. In both diagnosis and treatment, the machine was still junior partner to the doctor. By the time my father qualified as a doctor in Cape Town in 1939, the situation had changed again, and from then on until today doctor, patient and machine have all become increasingly intertwined with one another in an uncomfortable *ménage a trois*.

Actually, you could trace this process much further back, to Laennec's invention of the stethoscope in 1818. To the medical historian Roy Porter this was 'the most important diagnostic innovation before the discovery of X-rays in the 1890s.' Originally just a tube 23 cm long, Laennec's invention made it possible to hear a very different set of messages from the patient. For the first time doctors could identify, and localise, a diseased part of the body, in a way never possible before. They could actually examine a diseased organ separately from the person who contained it. By 1852 two ear-pieces had been added by the American physician George P. Cammann, and the stethoscope took on its present form. Draped around the neck like the two-headed serpent of Aesculapius, it has become the true badge of the modern doctor, one of medicine's most potent 'ritual symbols'. Even as a child I remember the curious power of this serpentine object, as I played reverentially with my father's stethoscope, with its heavy rubber tubes, gleaming silver frame, and the dark end-piece, heavy and black.

With the aid of this device, the body now 'speaks' directly to the doctor. And it tells its own particular tale. To make a diagnosis, you no longer have to listen quite so closely to what the ill person says. More important than the 'history' these days is the body's own narrative, decoded by diagnostic devices and the many new-fangled diagnostic machines. Often it's a narrative of numbers, easier to understand, easier to interpret, and easier, too, to arrange billing for. All of this represents a major shift over time from the person to the machine, from the subjective to the objective.

Sometime in the past century or so, subtly and without fanfare, the sign has become more important to doctors than the symptom.

Today the body speaks to the doctor mainly in a tremulous electronic whisper. On its way to the doctor, its voice passes through one complex machine after another. The electrocardiogram inscribes the wiggly electrical signature of its heart, the electroencephalogram that of its brain, the electromyograph that of the muscles. And ever since the X-ray machine was invented in 1895, the body's borders of skin have been dissolved. Since then the body has been transparent to the gaze of a medical machine. With the aid of CAT scans or MRIs, as well as X-rays, the doctor can now 'enter' the body and see all its secrets without having to cut open its envelope of skin.

Increasingly, these diagnostic messages bypass the patients themselves. After all, who knows more about the interior of their stomachs or lungs – the patient or the endoscopy tube? The person or the X-ray machine? But as doctors learn more about the body, they seem to listen to what their patients say much less. That's why Oliver Sacks's detailed narratives of his neurological patients and Richard Selzer's stories of his surgical patients, are so unusual, and so welcome. For in the rushed world of hospital clinics and wards, few doctors today have the time to listen to their patients any more, and hardly any have the interest. Thanks to medical technology, it's the patients' own personal 'histories' that have gradually receded, to be replaced by the narratives of their bodies.

Whirring and pulsing beside the patient's bed in the ward stands a large rectangular machine, all its surfaces shiny and metallic. Emerging from it are wires in red and blue coils and long silver spirals, many of them connected to the patient's body. Along its edges are numerous shiny screws and bolts, and rows of tiny rivets. This machine has illuminated dials and several green luminescent screens that glow in the dark. And it speaks in a strange, repetitive language: *bip-bip-bip-bip-bip*, it says. Or sometimes *Beeeeeeeep*!! That particular long sound always has a dramatic effect, causing a small crowd of doctors and nurses to run wildly into the ward, shouting to one another, and wheeling in another machine: a defibrillator. One machine has called to another for help – and that call is being swiftly answered.

Just as machines like this have become a sort of 'doctor', so has the patient's body increasingly become seen as a type of malfunctioning 'machine'. But according to Roy Porter, this concept of the body-as-machine is not at all new, for it actually emerged much earlier, as part of the Scientific Revolution of the 17th century, with its view of universal laws governing a clockwork world. From Descartes onwards, the body was seen primarily as a mechanical object: its heart a type of pump, its limbs just levers of bone and muscle, its diseases due mainly to mechanical breakdown.

Since then, writes Porter, there have also been other fundamental changes, for we now also tend to explain 'the whole in terms of its parts, the complex in terms of the simple, the biological in terms of the physical or chemical.' As a result, 'the core medical project over the past two centuries has lain in exploring the workings and the malfunctions of bodily tissues and cells.' But not, it seems, in a deeper understanding of the patient's belief system or point of view.

Even the prestigious *Journal of the American Medical Association* has sounded a warning bell. It saw the US medical system becoming so impersonal, so dominated by technology, that in an editorial in 1983 it felt obliged to ask the question: 'Has the machine become the physician?' 'The fact that the health care provided in the system may be improved as a result of the technology', wrote *JAMA*, 'does not have as much impact as the subtle and hidden message that the machine has become the physician: the definitive adviser. The specialist-physician is metamorphosing into a technocrat and a businessman. The physician retreats behind the machine, and becomes an extension of the machine.'

In many of today's high-tech hospitals, human patients must now compete for attention with paper patients. These new 'patients' are mostly thin and pale. They lie quietly wherever they are put. They are easy to control and easy to measure. They are clear and largely unambiguous. And unlike most human patients, they never complain, never answer back – and they definitely never sue. That is why some doctors seem to prefer them to the real thing. This new group of patients are the offspring of diagnostic technology: its printouts of blood tests, charts of vital signs, reports of X-rays and ultrasound scans, measurements of height, weight or pulmonary function. Nestling in the patients' folders or displayed at the foot of their beds, these 'paper patients' sometimes attract more detailed care and attention than the frightened people lying in the bed before them.

Picture the scene. Holding up the strip of electrocardiogram paper before him, the Professor turns to his entourage of junior staff and medical students. He speaks to them briefly in an unknown tongue:

'As you can see,' he says, ' although the heart is in sinus rhythm, the T- wave is slightly inverted, especially in Leads II and III, and the PR interval is definitely increased.'

('The tea wave?' wonders the patient, 'What does he mean? Does tea have *waves*? In a cup? What has this to do with me? And with my heart? And what is this 'PR' interval? Does he mean Public Relations? How can you tell all of that from just that little piece of paper?').

These paper patients are part, not only of our medical system, but of the paradox of modern society itself, the way it pays lip service to individualism, while at the same time reducing individuals themselves to standardised, impersonal, disposable entities.

Together with all their whirring and expensive machines, their statistics and pocket calculators, a new generation of sleek young men and women in smart white coats has emerged. They are clever and efficient, but the problem is – as so many patients have complained to me – there's something detached, almost robotic about some of them. It's as if some (hopefully only a small minority) have become the servants of the machines, instead of their masters. I call these people: *techno-doctors.*

As hospitals have gradually become temples to the Medical Machine, so these techno-doctors have become the High Priests of this new religion. Often they are super-specialists, experts on only one tiny bit of the body but not on the rest. They tend to be the doctors who study, in greatest detail, only shards or fragments of their patients. It's like an archaeology of the living: indispensable and useful, but also limited.

This specialisation has been the blessing of medicine, but also its curse. It has led to enormous medical and surgical advances over the years, but for many doctors it has also led to a certain narrowing of vision, an over-focus on the part rather than on the whole. And this process has been increasing steadily ever since the end of the 19th century, until today it dominates almost all of medical practice. A century ago, 90 per cent of American doctors would have described themselves as 'generalists'. Now only 12 per cent are in general or family practice. In the USA there are now no less than 41 medical specialties, and 25 sub-specialities.

Many of this new breed of specialist and techno-doctor have no time for family physicians or general practitioners, with their broad and unfocused areas of knowledge, their archaic listening skills, their collections of medical tales and quaint clinical aphorisms. And yet, to me, there is still something quietly heroic about most family doctors, with their huge workloads, over-crowded waiting-rooms and rushed consultation times. It's a solitary, un-rewarded type of heroism, far from the paparazzi and the public view, far from the expensive glitter of laboratories and all the other temples of Medical Science.

Family medicine – at least in Britain – is perhaps the last bastion of old-style medical holism, but even here it's still the Cinderella of medical specialties, way down on the medical food chain, far, far below the specialist techno-doctors. Yet despite everything, it still holds the personal, the subjective and the social to be important – especially the patients' own narratives of their illnesses, as well as their family 'history'. Sight and hearing and touch are still just as crucial as diagnostic machines. Despite being relatively low-tech, in Britain it is still the family doctors who are most often consulted by the public, the ones most engaged in human life, and with the raw mass of human suffering, the ones who work, every day of the week, with all the ambiguities of human life and suffering.

Techno-medicine, by contrast, offers us a dream of a world without ambiguity, of a scientific paradise in which everything makes sense, one where almost everything can be measured and then translated into the language of numbers. It's a utopia where Science replaces spirituality, and uncertainty has no place, where the patient's emotions, fears and belief system and spirituality are less important than the printout from a diagnostic machine, where the body in hospital is an imperfect machine and not part of a questioning person. But it's a fantasy, an intellectual cul-de-sac. For in real life the body is not everything, and – as I've learned again and again, over the years – both ambiguity and uncertainty will always be part of any form of medical practice.

As the cancer specialist Rachel Nancy Remen has put it: 'Perhaps the most basic skill of the physician is the ability to have comfort with uncertainty, to recognise with humility the uncertainty inherent in all situations, to be open to the ever-present possibility of the surprising, the mysterious, and even the holy, and to meet people there.'

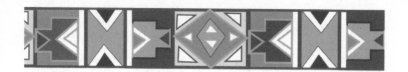

CHAPTER
21

Shamans

Elias is short and stocky, with a strong face. He has a convinced, emphatic manner, and when he speaks he makes chopping or pointing movements with his powerful hands. He is shrewd and charismatic and strong. With his whitening beard, his long red cloak and beaded head-dress, a tattered and coverless Bible in one hand, a fly whisk in another, he reminds me somehow of an Old Testament prophet. And in fact, that is close to the pivotal role he plays within his own community. Now he stands barefoot before me on the dusty floor of his thatched mud hut, while his wife sits on a wooden stool in one corner, and the interpreter and I sit on a long bench in the other. Standing in the shadowy centre of the hut, Elias throws a piece of springbok hide down onto the floor, and then steps onto it. He points at it, then at the Bible, then at the fly whisk.

'He says, "These are my stethoscopes,"'says the interpreter. 'He says to tell you that this is how he finds out what is wrong with people. He stands on it and then *izinyanya*, the spirits of his ancestors, speak to him and tell him what is the problem.'

Elias is a *sangoma*, a traditional Xhosa healer in a remote area of the

Transkei, in the Eastern Cape region of South Africa. Most doctors despise people like Elias. They see them as quacks and charlatans and 'witch doctors', though they are neither witches nor doctors. They see the treatments and advice that they give as unscientific, irrational and often dangerous. They point out that you cannot see Elias's ancestral spirits on a microscope slide, nor measure their effects with a blood test or CAT scan, that there is no scientific evidence that any of his treatments work.

For his community, however, Elias functions rather like any family doctor: as the first line of defence and explanation, when people feel ill or unhappy. He is a type of 'shaman', a traditional healer who, under certain circumstances, can incarnate spirits or gods. Often in a state of trance, and with the aid of these spirits and his 'stethoscopes', he can diagnose the causes of illness and tell the victim how they should be dealt with. For all his lack of scientific knowledge, he has all the skills of a shrewd psychotherapist and a clever social worker, combined with those of a religious exorcist. As the anthropologist I. M. Lewis puts it 'The shaman is not less than a psychiatrist, he is more.'

A shaman is often called a 'master of spirits' (though many of them are female), or a 'god box' – as one of the Polynesian languages puts it. Like mediums or channellers, they see themselves as merely the conduit of forces much greater than themselves, of something that flows through them and then into their words and their actions. Many artists I know also feel this. Once I met a potter in Finland, a mystical man, and asked him how he signed his work. He showed me the small metal die, with his initials engraved on it, that he stamped into the clay before it was fired.

'But if I produce something *very* beautiful, something *very* wonderful,' he adds, 'then of course I would never sign it.'

'Why not?' I ask.

He shrugs. 'Because then obviously it's not mine any more'.

'Ask Elias what is the most common thing wrong with people in this area,' I say to the interpreter. 'What do they mostly come to see him about?'

Elias taps his forehead, smiles, rolls his eyes, shakes his head. The beads swirl around his face, like chains of random thought.

'Mad,' he says in English, 'mad!' And then more in Xhosa.

'He says people who are mad,' the interpreter tells me, 'mad up here. Crazy.'

He describes some of the different causes of 'mad', from 'thinking too much', to 'witchcraft' from other people and 'water on the brain'. Whatever the cause, the results are roughly similar: depression, worries, insomnia, conflicts between husbands and wives, parents and children. Ask any family doctor in Britain the same question, and the Usual Suspects would be roughly the same – that large group of patients known as 'the worried well'. But in this setting the shaman's job, like that of any healer, is to give meaning to his clients' suffering, to give it shape and form, to impose order on the random chaos of personal misfortune. Above all to help them make sense of what has happened and why.

Shamans are wounded people. Becoming one, like becoming a doctor, is not easy. Sometimes it can even destroy them. Often it all begins with a major crisis. Possessed by the gods or their ancestral spirits, they can become seriously ill in their body or go crazy in their mind. It can be a painful, terrifying experience, one that few ever welcome. And in the Transkei, once they've suffered possession, they can go one of two ways. It can be *amafafunyana*, and the spirits master them, and their dark fate will then be madness, disease or death. Or it can be *ukuthwasa*, in which they master the spirits and so follow the call of their ancestors to become a sangoma. Once a true 'master of spirits' they can, with their help, diagnose and heal others. Like a psychoanalyst, they have undergone a long ritual of personal healing. 'The shaman,' wrote Mircea Eliade, 'is not only a sick man; he is above all, a sick man who has been cured, who has succeeded in curing himself.'

Shamans at work, particularly in a trance, would look quite 'mad' to any psychiatrist. Watching movies of them at work gives the same impression. Technically, they do have some of the characteristics of the psychotic: a 'loss of self identity', 'hearing voices' and a certain lack of psychic boundaries, enabling them to 'share' thoughts and emotions with their clients or with invisible spirits. But shamans are not mad. Their behaviour is not random, but controlled and patterned by the culture in which they live. Their trances happen in ways, and at times, that make sense to their communities, who in turn welcome this brief glimpse into that numinous Other World, the one unbounded by time and space, that the shaman brings to them.

The apparent 'madness' of shamanism – really a misinterpretation by Western observers – reminds me of the wry remark, attributed to Salvador Dali. 'The only difference between me and a madman,' he's supposed to have said, 'is that I am *not* mad.'

During their training, it's quite common for shamans to have dreams or visions of fragmentation and dismemberment. Bits of their body are separated from each other, limbs scattered wide apart, organs eaten by invisible spirits. Sometimes this happens as part of some hallucinogenic trance, though not always. But shamans are not the only healers who suffer this fate and who have to become wounded as part of their education. In our society, too, doctors are subtly 'disassembled' as part of their training. But this seems to take place in a very different way – outside their bodies, and in the bodies and psyches of other people rather than in their own. It happens in the dismantling of cadavers in the dissecting room, or in the autopsies in the Pathology Department. Every day the silver scalpels are dismantling not only a dead person, but also something within the students themselves, some sense of the inherent unity and coherence of the human body and of the human self, of the sense of being more than just the sum of one's parts. Dissecting others, they are, one could say, actually dissecting themselves.

Even if they're not emotionally wounded by dissection and autopsies and the daily exposure to human suffering as a student, then they have to face the long hours and stressful intensity of the internship and residency years. And if they weren't wounded before, then this will surely do the job.

And much later, working in clinical practice, the doctors (like shamans or psychoanalysts) will have to first master their own inner demons, whether personal or professional, before trying to master those of others. And many will spend much of their professional lives trying unsuccessfully to re-assemble this coherent image of the human, to put the Humpty-Dumpty of the patient – and of themselves – back together again.

What can we learn from people like Elias? From the scientific techno-doctors, the simple answer is: Nothing. Absolutely nothing. But I disagree. And so does the World Health Organisation. Back in 1978 it first recognised their value, especially in areas where doctors are few. They saw the advantage of traditional medicine as lying in its 'holistic approach – i.e., that of viewing man in his totality within a wide ecological spectrum, and of emphasising the viewpoint that ill health or disease is brought about by an imbalance, or disequilibrium, of man in his total ecological system, and not only by the causative agent and pathogenic evolution.'

The WHO saw traditional healers as possible allies of the medical system, not necessarily as its opponents. They regarded them as gifted and experienced folk psychologists, local 'social workers', community and religious leaders, experts on local herbs and on other remedies and healing techniques. 'Get them on your side', was the message, especially in preventing AIDS, improving child health, in family planning programmes, and in dealing with mental health problems within a community. In all of this debate though, it is also important not to over-romanticise them, to be cautious about their superstitious beliefs and practices, and the dangers these may sometimes pose. But overall, the belief is that they can still be useful. In many parts of the world now, they even work in co-operation with doctors, as on the Navaho Reservation in south-western USA.

For many traditional practitioners (including those in Traditional Chinese Medicine, and in Indian Ayurveda) really are as holistic as WHO says they are. One thing that we can learn from them is the way they see health as *balance*, as a state of equilibrium, not only within a person's body and psyche, but also in that person's relationships with the other people around them, with the natural environment, and with the world of their gods or ancestral spirits. To them, sickness, bad luck, even death, are all signs of an imbalance in any of these relationships – and the aim of the healer is to restore that balance. As with old-fashioned medicine – before the recent rise of the techno-doctors – it's a view of illness that takes it outside the body, its diseased organs and the purely physical, and then places it in its wider personal, social and cosmic context. Whatever else is going on in their lives, for people and healers in these communities, health is harmony – and illness not just the malfunction of a particular organ.

I ask Elias about AIDS and his attitude towards it. He says that he's heard of it, but that he doesn't really know what it is. He says that he doesn't really believe it exists. But what he does know for sure, he says, is that if a man sleeps around with lots of women who are not his wife – or if a woman sleeps with men who are not her husband – then they will often get ill. They will sicken, get thin and weak, and eventually die. With such illicit relationships, there is no such thing as 'safe sex'. He blames this on their ancestors punishing them for their immoral behaviour. Perhaps the doctors can help them then, but he can do nothing. It's too late for that. Now it's the doctors' turn.

To Western ears, his model is harsh and moralistic. But in terms of preventing AIDS, by changing behaviour, he and the doctors agree. And maybe in the future they can even work together.

Elias works in a poor, rural environment, in which much of the belief system is summed up by the well-known Xhosa saying: *Ubuntu ngumntu ngabanye abantu* ('People are people through other people'). Each person's humanity is expressed through a relationship with others, and their humanity in turn comes through a recognition of his or hers. To be uninvolved with other people, and in the life of the community, is to be an incomplete person.

As practitioners of this view, people like Elias are essential to the continuity and cohesion of their communities, and their emotional well-being, in a way that Western doctors never are. It's also a community where, as in much of sub-Saharan Africa, the dead never die. For the ancestors remain in the world of the living as invisible guardians of the moral order, punishing their descendants with illness, madness or death if they ever step out of line. In a traditional society like this, nothing is arbitrary. As interpreted by the traditional healer, all things make sense, especially disease. In each case the victim and their family may wonder: 'What have I done?' 'Whom have I offended?' Or even: 'Who has done this to me?' And it's only people like Elias who can give them the answers.

In his studies of traditional healing, published in the 1960s, Victor Turner describes another shaman, the *chimbuki* or traditional healer of the Ndembu people of Zambia. In this group, many believe that all serious illness is caused by conflict between people, as well as by witchcraft or the punishments of ancestral spirits – and thus the healer has to deal with illness in a very special way. Gathering the family or community together when someone falls ill, he asks them to declare their grudges publicly against the victim, while in turn the victim must acknowledge his grudges against them. By bringing family, friends and neighbours together around the patient, and then by airing – and resolving – all the hidden conflicts between them, he is not only healing the individual, but also the group, restoring relationships, soothing their troubled minds, relaxing their troubled bodies.

Even in our Western setting, remarks Turner, 'relief might be given to many sufferers from neurotic illness if all those involved in their social networks could meet together and publicly confess their ill will towards the patient, and endure in turn the recital of his grudges against them.'

Part social worker, part family therapist, part priest, the *chimbuki* (like Elias the sangoma) may certainly not be able to cure tuberculosis, heart disease, a tumour or AIDS. But he can make people feel better and even improve their relationships with others. Unlike many of today's scientific techno-doctors, the *chimbuki* can heal, even if he cannot cure.

Gallup, New Mexico is an upside-down sort of place, where cowboys and Indians appear to have changed places. As I stroll up the main street young Navaho men gallop past me on piebald ponies wearing stetsons and high-heeled boots, while white people crowd the sidewalks, dripping with turquoise and silver Indian jewellery. Driving out of town, I visit a Navaho friend on the Reservation, not far from Lukachukai, to talk about another type of healing. Over coffee and crackers in her office in a circular building, based on a traditional *hogan*, I tell her how, back in London, I often get so tired and exhausted (I could have added 'angry, depressed, frustrated') after seeing so many patients in a day. She nods sympathetically. That is the fate of all healers. She tells me that her grandfather was a Navaho traditional healer, and that he, too, often came back emotionally drained from doing his healing ceremonies or 'sings' – some of which took several days to perform. But then that he, and his family, dealt with this in a very different way. Each time he returned, she tells me, her grandmother would take over the healing role, performing special rituals and songs for him, so that the wounded healer would now become healed in his turn.

'And my grandfather always said that if you felt like that, you should always stroke a horse,' she adds, 'or a newborn baby. Both of them are so full of energy. You will feel much better if you touch them, straight-away.'

But unfortunately for me, I cannot take her advice, for the baby has long grown into adulthood, and horses to stroke are in short supply in my part of suburban London.

Porto Alegre – a small industrial city with many high-rise buildings, on the banks of the Guaiba River – is the southernmost city in Brazil, in the state of Rio Grande do Sul. Like other Brazilian cities, it has a parallel world of poverty and sprawling shantytowns, or *favelas*. There is also a parallel world of belief and superstition, and a proliferation of new religions. One evening in the early 1990s, together with two Brazilian anthropologists, I am taken to attend one of the *sessões*, or religious ceremonies of Umbanda, a fairly new and syncretic Brazilian religion that mingles popular Catholicism with native Brazilian and West African elements into a heady and popular mixture. It's a type of collective healing ceremony, a mixture of religion, dance, group thera-py and personal catharsis. They warn me that during the ceremony, some people will become 'possessed', and look quite 'crazy'.

It takes place in a *centro*, a small building hidden in the yard behind a larger one, much like the servant's quarters of a big house in Johannesburg. The place is already buzzing, filled with crowds of peo-ple in long black, white or red cloaks, or even turbans, milling around. On a small platform on one side sits a small group of drummers, warming up. On a high altar on the other side are displayed the massed and mingled gods of Umbanda, a bright-coloured collection of wood or painted plaster. They include the *Orixas* – a poetic pantheon mainly West African in origin, among whom are *Iamanjá*, Goddess of the Sea; *Iansã*, Goddess of the Wind; *Oxum*, Goddess of Fresh Waters; *Oxum-Manre*, the Goddess of Rainbows; *Ogum*, God of War; *Xangô*, like Thor, God of Thunder and Lightning; and *Oxôssi*, skilful hunter of the forests. And then there are the *Caboclos*, the spirits of indigenous Brazilian Indians, in their big feathered head-dresses; and the *Pretos Velhos*, spirits of old black slaves, long deceased; and a wide selection of familiar Catholic saints: St Michael, St George, St Jerome, and the rest. It's a huge population of helpful gods, as diverse and colourful as the people of Brazil themselves.

Now the drumming is intensifying into a rhythmic, hypnotic beat. I can feel myself beginning to sway, and move with the music. A bottle of some powerful liquid is passed around, and many are swigging from it, but I decline. There's no need for it, for already I feel intoxicated. My head is spinning as the dancers swirl swiftly around us, circling and swaying as they become possessed, many bent forward and walking slowly backwards, their arms dangling down before them.

At the edges of the room, I notice that whispered consultations (*consultas*) are now beginning to take place between officiants in white robes and dancers who have drifted, one by one, towards them. Each officiant has now become a medium, possessed by a different deity. Through them the clients are consulting these spirits, asking them for help, healing or advice. Many have come to have their own evil spirits exorcised by the mediums. Others have come for absolution. My friends point out which mediums have become possessed by which gods or spirits. You can tell it from their voices, their movements and posture – from the wild restless movements and shrill cries of the *Caboclos*, with their stern faces, to the slow, shambling, unsteady gait of the elderly *Pretos Velhos*, puffing on their invisible pipes.

Round and round us the people swirl, the drums beat faster every moment. People are possessed, exorcised, possessed again, eyes rolling, their bodies contorted by this cosmic struggle.

Hours pass, a timeless blur of dance and drum. And much, much later in the evening when the dancing has finally slowed and the musicians have begun packing up their drums, and the sky outside is velvet and speckled with stars, I look around me. The room is subdued, the people drifting home quietly. They look relaxed now, content, much calmer than before. Their lives in the ramshackle *favelas* around us are difficult and uncertain as always, but at least for now they feel a little better. A type of collective healing has taken place. It hasn't helped their economic woes, but for one evening, at least, they can become a god, or else consult with a god or a spirit, the incarnation of something much greater than themselves. They can dance and whirl, and be touched and listened to intently by important people. They can if they wish be exorcised, and in front of everyone fall writhing to the floor, in a wild, ecstatic, unforgettable catharsis. But at the end of the evening, they all know that they will go home feeling better, or even happy.

On another visit to Porto Alegre, a year later, a colleague and I are introduced to Dona Maria, a *Mae de Santo* – or Mother of Saints. She is the high priestess of another *centro*, and also a healer. In the empty hall built beside her home, Donna Maria sits opposite us with her own vast array of gods watching us silently from behind her, and does a divination for me. For a moment she looks distant, dreamy, far away. Then suddenly she throws her collection of bones, shells, and pieces of wood down onto the little table between us. She stares at them intently for a long while. Then, like a tarot reader, she tells me about myself (most things accurate, a few not), and then the name of my personal patron saint (St Michael, I think). More significantly, she tells us how she works with the sick people who consult her, how she frequently refers them back to the doctors and nurses at the local clinic, if they are seriously ill. Like Elias in the Transkei and the Navaho healers, her approach is surprisingly pragmatic. Unlike many doctors I know, she seems to realise the limits of her own expertise – which conditions she can treat and which she cannot.

Like most other traditional healers (as well as priests and religious figures) Dona Maria specialises in answering the *why?* questions, the ones that always crop up when people fall unexpectedly ill. 'Why has it happened?' they ask.' Why to *me*? Why *now*?' Or, 'What have I done to deserve it?'

For their part, medical doctors seem to specialise more in the *what?* questions. They explain to their patients, precisely and scientifically, exactly what has happened – that their coronary vessels have clogged up, that their pancreas has not been producing enough insulin, or that their leg has been broken in two different places.

'Yes, but *why*?' asks the patient, 'why did it happen then? Who did it to me? Did I offend the gods?'

On this, the doctors are silent. That's where Dona Maria comes in, placing the event in a wider framework, one of human relationships or of relations with the divine. When they go home from her *centro*, her clients carry with them a special gift: a story of their suffering, carefully crafted, explaining why it ever happened. Like the *chimbuki* and Elias, Dona Maria can often heal their minds, and their relationships, even if she cannot cure their bodies.

I have always been interested in folk healing and in traditional forms of health care, and in their advantages and disadvantages, but that interest doesn't come from nowhere. In the summer of 1993 I have the opportunity to visit the village or *shtetl* along the Baltic coast, where my own ancestor, a folk practitioner, once lived – the first in our long medical line. Now it is a small market town, set beside endless wheat fields and dense forests of pine, beech and fir, on the banks of a winding river. Here is where my great-great-great-grandfather was born in 1802, and where he, and two of his sons were *feldshers* – not shamans, but village practitioners or barber-surgeons.

In the Russian Empire of the 18th and 19th centuries, people like them were a sort of proto-general practitioner – the only source of medical treatment available to poor, rural communities. Originally founded by Peter the Great in the 18th century, many of the *feldshers* were ex-army medics sent out to work in the villages once their service was over. There were doctors in the large towns and cities, of course, but they were distant and expensive. By the 20th century, the former Soviet Union had incorporated all the *feldshers* into its medical system as 'physician-assistants' – lower-grade practitioners, handmaidens now of the 'real' doctors.

In *Baptism by Rotation*, a story from his *A Country Doctor's Notebook*, Mikhail Bulgakov describes his encounter with a difficult birth, in the winter darkness of a remote rural village. In delivering the baby he is aided not only by the nurse, but also by one Demyan Lukich, the local *feldsher*. In Dr Bulgakov's day, during the First World War, practitioners like Demyan had already become much less than a doctor, but also much more than a nurse.

In that summer of 1993, together with the Lithuanian poet and journalist, Rimantas Vanagas, I visit my ancestor's town, where Vanagas's family also originate. He shows me the Roman Catholic cathedral, with its twin spires of red brick, on the banks of the river, the Old Town with its tilting brick and wooden houses, the ancient Catholic and Jewish cemeteries, the various war graves, the Holocaust site deep in the forest (3000 people murdered here in 1941, on one day), and the squat sprawling modernity of the Soviet-era housing.

Standing at the river's edge – while laden barges drift slowly by me in the warm summer breeze – I think of my great-great-great grandfather travelling around here almost two centuries ago, among the cornfields and the little wooden houses, by foot or in horse-and-buggy, setting bones, pulling teeth, treating the ailments of the peasants and the local Jewish community with his leeches and cups, his herbal concoctions and cabbage leaf dressings.

A man who spanned two traditions – part medical practitioner, part traditional folk healer.

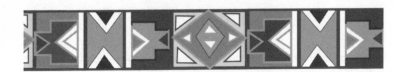

CHAPTER
22

Placebos

The Medical Rep sits across from me, a young man with a smart blue suit and a big briefcase. He has slicked black hair, every strand carefully in place. He smiles like Father Christmas as he opens his briefcase and hands out free gifts of ballpoint pens, calendars, paperweights and little plastic souvenirs, each one stamped with his company's logo in bright red letters along its side.

Today he is trying to promote 'X', a newish drug for reducing stomach acid and helping to heal and prevent stomach ulcers. He shows me a large laminated card with some research findings printed on it. There are two groups of people with stomach ulcers: one has been given 'X', his company's drug, the other an inactive look-alike, an exact copy but really just a sugar pill, a placebo. With his carefully manicured finger he points to two big numbers at the bottom of the card: one in green, the other in black. He points particularly at the green number, jabbing at the card several times.

'As you can see here, Doctor, 75 per cent of the group given 'X' had their stomach ulcers completely healed after only six weeks of treatment – but only 41 per cent were healed by the placebo!'

It's impressive, I agree. I don't say anything as he leaves, smiling, but what *really* impresses me is the fact that 41 per cent of a group of people can have their ulcers completely healed by a piece of sugar. Just by the power of their belief. To me it's extraordinary. For that is the placebo effect, and in medical practice it's a very powerful and mysterious thing.

Over the years, it's always seemed odd to me the way that medical journals and textbooks (and Medical Reps) sneer at the placebo effect. The way that they dismiss it as 'only the placebo effect', or 'just a placebo' – as if it were something unreal, immaterial and quite irrelevant, an epiphenomenon of the real tasks of scientific medicine.

Why is this so? Perhaps, to the more rigid medical mind, placebos really are an embarrassment, a ghost at the medical feast. For they seem to represent effects on the body that, from a scientific point of view, cannot easily be explained, nor easily predicted. They are the weak link in the scientific medical paradigm, the point at which its power, and its powers of explanation, are limited. It is that part of the healing process contributed by the patient's own psyche as well as their body.

And yet, everything I've read in both anthropology and medical history tells me that, worldwide, most healers (and most doctors) have always had a very different view of this phenomenon. They know it works, and that you should never ignore the powers of suggestion. They regard the placebo effect as an ally in healing, and not as an enemy, and thus strive to enhance it in every way. Of course, scattered among these healers is the usual quota of quacks or charlatans, but in general a positive attitude towards the patient's belief system seems to be true of every type of healer, in every age and in all human societies – though increasingly less so, it seems, in our own.

Maybe that's one of the greatest differences between traditional healers (such as shamans) and many modern doctors, and between doctors and many of the new alternative healers. Increasingly, medicine focuses mainly on pathology, on the diseases and disorders of the patient's body as revealed by diagnostic technology. It focuses less on their healthy parts, their personality, their own inner resources, psychological as well as physical, the sorts of invisible strengths that simply don't show up on a CAT scan or an X-ray plate. It's what high-tech medical diagnosis and treatment is increasingly about – the detailed, often microscopic examination of diseased organs and bodily systems. But this approach can sometimes turn the patient into a victim, and their body into a passive battlefield between microbes or diseases on one side, and surgery and drugs on the other.

In contrast to this, many traditional healers and alternative practitioners tend to focus more on *health*, as much as on disease. Their aim is to build up their patients' active strength – physical, psychological, social and even spiritual – to help them fight the affliction and to prevent any recurrences of it. That's why they try always to increase their patient's faith not only in the healer, but also in themselves, and to get them actively on their side. They strive to convince them of how, in association with the healer, they can help fight the disease, whether by following certain rituals or certain diets, or even by saying certain prayers. These are all things that they *do* – not that are done to them.

A friend of mine, a diabetologist who works among a small Native American population in the USA, has told me how his diabetic patients often ignore his advice and warnings if they are couched in a negative way. 'Watch your diet, and take more exercise, or you'll go into diabetic coma, or your nerves will be damaged, or your heart will fail, or some of your limbs may even have to be amputated.' Spoken to in those terms, his patients often switch off and withdraw. But if he puts the advice in another, more positive way, the result – he says – is often very different: 'Watch your diet, and take more exercise, because then you'll be strong, and more healthy, and you'll feel well, and happier, and you'll have more energy and fewer health problems, and both you and your family will have a much better life.' It's a subtle difference in approach, but an important one. To appeal always to the positive, to the healthy, functioning, hopeful part of sick people – and not just to their pathology. In this way you make them your active ally in the management of their disease. The first approach turns the patients into fearful victims, the second into active participants, people who believe in themselves and their own powers to alleviate their diseases.

Despite the scornful attitudes of the medical journals, it should be said that in practice most doctors also try to enhance belief in a similar way, and have always done so, but they call it something else: 'achieving rapport', 'good bedside manner' or 'good doctor-patient communication'. And it still is (or should be) an important part of any medical education.

Way back at the very beginning of Western medical history, Hippocrates knew all about it, too, and how important it was for patients to maintain a deep faith in their physicians. He knew the power of mind over body. 'Some patients, though concerned that their condition is perilous, recover their health simply through their contentment with the goodness of their physician,' he wrote over two millennia ago. With the aid of that trust, the physician could use the patient's own natural processes as vital allies in the treatment. And it's as true today as it was then.

The more time I spend in clinical practice, and the more I learn about the powers of belief, the stranger seem the tricks that the mind can play on the body, stranger even than the 41 per cent with their healed-up stomach ulcers, as proved by endoscopy and X-ray. Medical (and psychiatric) textbooks are full of examples of this, as is daily clinical experience. Many of these cases are examples not of the placebo effect, but of its opposite – what has been called the 'nocebo' effect. This refers to the negative consequence of belief, in which a belief or a suggestion (or even the attitudes of other people) can make you feel unwell, or anxious or depressed, or damage your health in other ways. In some rare cases it can even kill you. The most extreme example of this, reported by anthropologists from several tribal societies, has been called 'voodoo death'. Here, in a public ritual of accusation, a powerful sorcerer or religious figure puts a curse on a particular individual, as punishment for breaking some important rule or taboo. Soon everyone in the tribe withdraws from the doomed man, ignoring him, refusing to speak to him, looking right through him – as if he were already dead. And soon he actually does die – often within a day or two – apparently of natural causes. A victim of the powers of suggestion.

But medical practice is full of much less dramatic examples of the nocebo effect, and its effect on body and mind. Take, for example, *pseudocyesis*, a rare condition I've only read about, but never actually seen. Apparently it's a type of phantom pregnancy that occurs in some women who yearn to be pregnant, but who for some reason cannot conceive or who are are nearing menopause. For these women, it's their Last Chance Saloon. And then something happens to them, but at a very deep unconscious level. They become absolutely convinced that they are pregnant, whatever anyone else may say. Soon they actually develop many of the physical changes of normal pregnancy. Their periods stop, they put on weight, their bellies swell up, their breasts enlarge and sometimes even secrete milk. They may develop morning sickness, imagine fetal movements within their uterus, even the onset of labour pains. They can have every symptom of pregnancy, but without actually being pregnant. In physiological terms, this rare condition is apparently due to unusual hormonal changes involving the pituitary gland. But pseudocyesis is also one of the most powerful examples I know of mind over matter, of how a hope or a delusion (or a belief) can actually sculpt a human body from within, as it were, into its very own shape and form.

To a large extent, it's obvious that placebo effects are part of every type of healing, whether medical or not. Anthropologists have reported them from all over the world. But when you look at them more closely, you can see that most forms of healing are also theatrical performances designed to enhance this effect. Just like other forms of theatre, they use props, costumes, sets and a precise choreography to achieve this effect. But of course it's theatre with a serious intent, and not just for entertainment. Its aim is to help the process of healing along by creating a certain atmosphere of belief and expectation, a milieu that encourages confidence in the patient's mind. Even my own consulting room, when I come to think about it, can be seen as a type of stage-set within which, each day, a dozen or so small human dramas are played out. It, too, has its props and its scenery, its backdrop and costumes, to create an effect, and even the choreography of most consultations is tightly scripted in advance. On this tiny stage, I find myself playing different roles at different times: sometimes a villain, often a hero, occasionally just a spectator.

The room has taken on its present form slowly over the years, and not by any conscious design. Against one wall stands a bookcase of impressive-looking medical textbooks (several out of date and rarely consulted), their thick spines lettered in fading silver or gold. Against another wall is a glass cabinet filled with row upon row of glittering silver instruments (some rarely used). There is an examination couch at one end, covered in clean white paper, behind a rattan screen. There are calendars from pharmaceutical companies hung on the walls, and a few coloured prints. There's a desk, a weighing machine, some charts on the wall, and a sink with clean towels draped beside it. In the air, like wafting incense in a holy shrine, you can inhale just the faintest tang of antiseptic.

Around the edge of my desk there is a Berlin Wall of objects that I have gradually (and unconsciously) erected between me and Them: two piles of patients' notes, and one of still-unread medical journals; a calendar or two; a family photograph; a blood pressure machine; an ophthalmoscope; a peak-flow meter; an oval container filled with wooden tongue spatulas; a holder for stationery and X-ray forms; a digital clock; and a yellow rubber heart, a gift from a pharmaceutical company, to squeeze vigorously whenever I get tense.

Early each morning, I sit in the same way and in the same place at the centre of this little stage, pen poised, formally costumed, my features arranged into a mask of focused compassion. 'First patient, please,' I call out.

The door opens. The curtain rises.

When you compare them, you can see that every healer's room – whether medical or not – gives the patient a different set of messages. Each one creates its own, unique version of the placebo effect. And in many of them the décor, furnishings, clothing, colour and smell – as well as the specific use of time and space – are not just background and setting, but are also actually part of the healing process itself. It's a situation where, as Marshall McLuhan once put it, the medium *is* the message. This is as true of a medical office or clinic as of the hut of a shaman or the holy shrine of a religious healer. Many of the objects that adorn its walls – whether pharmaceutical calendars, framed religious tracts, acupuncture charts, diagrams of bodily organs, rows of holy idols, crucifixes or even shelves full of scientific instruments – give powerful subliminal messages to the patient. To anthropologists, most of these items are not just neutral objects. They are what one writer has called 'multi-facetted mnemonics' – symbols that condense large amounts of information into them, telling the patients who the healer is, and what the true sources of his healing powers are. In that sense, looking around my room, I see myself as no different from any shaman or traditional healer. We come from different traditions, we have different frames of reference, but we both employ the same range of tricks to get our patients on our side.

My own consulting room in London is very different from the doctors' offices I've seen in the United States or Canada. They too have all the usual medical paraphernalia, but often these are 'framed' by a more glittering and flamboyant display of medical credentials. On the walls there are usually row upon row of diplomas and certificates, their impressive Latin calligraphy glassed and framed, and each one with a large seal in red, silver or gold. And next to them, often, a further display of citations, awards, photographs or even sports trophies. Like icons in a sacred shrine to the healing powers of Medical Science, the message of these massed diplomas is loud and emphatic: 'Look at me,' they say, 'I've studied, I've graduated, I've been licensed, I'm a success. Now *trust* me!'

By contrast, in the Freud Museum in North-West London, Sigmund Freud's consulting room, re-assembled in 1938 after his flight from Vienna, gives the client a very different set of messages. Most of the objects within it were brought along with him from Vienna, including his famous couch. Lying upon it, and free-associating, the analysand would have had a clear view of several shelves behind Freud's desk, crowded with the artefacts and figurines he had collected, mostly from ancient Greece, Rome and Egypt. This impressive display would clearly indicate to the client that Herr Professor Freud was particularly interested in the past, in the collective past, ancient and buried, but also in the patient's own individual past. And that is what they should be talking about. In this way, the décor of the room itself could be seen as an intrinsic part of the therapy, and it would echo Freud's own remark that the psychoanalyst's work 'resembles to a great extent an archaeologist's excavation of some dwelling-place that has been destroyed and buried.'

For many people, especially the frightened and the confused, much of the placebo effect lies in diagnosis as much as in treatment, for diagnosis is primarily order imposed upon chaos. It means finding a coherent pattern in the apparent disorder of an individual's suffering, and especially explaining to them why it has happened, why specifically to them, and why now. It's much the same process with healers everywhere: Dona Maria in Porto Alegre reading the diagnosis in the patterns of bones and shells; Elias in the Transkei divining the patterns of his ancestral dreams and voices; a psychotherapist in New York interpreting her client's chaotic jumble of dreams and emotions, and how they all fit together; and the family doctor in London, trying to place the specific pattern of a patient's symptoms, physical signs and changes in behaviour within a known diagnostic category.

For some patients then, diagnosis and treatment are not separate processes: diagnosis *is* treatment. The sense of order restored, at a time of great anxiety, is a powerful treatment in itself. As one Phineas Parkhurst Quimby, a famous folk healer born in New England in 1802, once put it, in an unconscious comment on the placebo effect:

'I tell the patient his troubles, and what he thinks is his disease, and my explanation is the cure. If I succeed in correcting his errors, I change the fluids in the system, and establish the patient in health. The truth is the cure.'

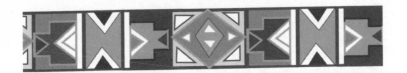

CHAPTER
23

Third Worlds

It's the 'Third World', but it could easily be the Fourth or the Fifth. The Transkei, birthplace of Nelson Mandela, is the poorest, most underdeveloped region of South Africa. As with Brazil and other parts of Latin America, you can see this poverty first on the outskirts of the towns, in the overcrowded shantytowns of corrugated iron, mud huts or tiny houses. There is often no heating or running water, no sewerage, electricity or telephones. Occasionally there is the luxury of a freshwater tap, or of a draughty dilapidated outhouse, but often not.

As some colleagues and I drive out from Umtata, the Transkei capital, the road changes. Tarmac becomes dirt road, then dirt road becomes rutted and winding track, meandering across the landscape. The four-wheeled drive sways and dips, like a schooner on rough seas. Clouds of reddish dust rise behind us. As we drive deeper into the veldt, most of the bluegum trees disappear. The land becomes drier, there are vistas of waving yellowed grass, a few shrubs or wildflowers, low hills of bleached khaki, a few blue mountains in the distance. Cracked river beds wander across our route, like thin dusty snakes searching for water. From time to time, small herds of goats or cows are driven across the road by shouting barefoot boys. Here and there are scattered clumps of homesteads – neat compounds of circular houses with thatched roofs, walls of sun-baked mud bricks painted in white or blue. A few chickens or tethered goats scratch around outside. The veldt is flat and dry, and endless. Above our heads, another endless space. The sky is vast and pellucid, a deep inverted ocean that goes on forever. As always in Africa, I feel only lightly held by the Earth's surface. The sky draws you up. I could easily float up into its infinite blueness.

We are heading for an old mission station, about an hour or so out of town. There's a small community health centre there, run in partnership by the provincial health department, the local community, and the University of Transkei Medical School. It's a low modest building of yellow-brown brick, with thick burglar-proof bars on every window. For only about eight hours each day, it's staffed by a dedicated team of two Cuban doctors and several African nurses, midwives, volunteers and security staff.

It's early morning, but already the waiting room is dense with people. Outside, another long line of people wait to be seen, while others sit in the waving grass, talking among themselves. Many of the women, with babies strapped to their backs, are wearing their traditional Xhosa garb: long dresses, headscarves tied into turbans, white clay smeared on their faces. I think of all my fretful patients back in London, glancing irritably at their watches, but here they are patient and quiet. Some cough into stained handkerchiefs. Others gently nurse a bandaged limb or try to comfort a fretful baby. A few of the women are breast-feeding. Many of these people have walked for hours across the veldt in order to get here.

Someone tells me that, together with a few tiny satellite clinics run by nurses, this health centre serves 60,000 people. It's difficult to believe. Sixty thousand people! For a moment I think I must have misheard, but no. And furthermore, after the clinic staff leave in the evening, there is nothing – no ambulances, no private doctors, only a few taxis, and a handful of public telephones scattered around. Until the next morning, there is only the indifferent veldt.

The health centre is spotless and well kept. There are several small consulting rooms, a wooden cupboard full of medications, and a maternity unit – three iron bedsteads in a tiny room, cows peering in through the windows. There's a new X-ray machine, but today there is no one to operate it. Resting on one reception counter is a 'Condoman Condotainer', a white box with a crossed red ribbon painted on one side. It's a free condom-dispenser, but while I'm watching, no one seems to take any. I wonder what the AIDS situation is in this area. Oscar, one of the Cubans, tells me that it's getting worse. The virus is out of control. It's spreading not only through the urban poor, but relentlessly through these rural communities as well. By the time they present themselves at the clinic, it's often too late. And drugs are in short supply (though this situation has recently improved). Often the disease comes in disguise, arriving as TB, shingles or a sudden loss in weight. A young man comes in only with shingles, and they hardly need to test him for HIV. Even before the test, they already suspect what he's got – and his wife, too, probably.

Many of the children die young – from infections, accidents, malnutrition, diarrhoeal diseases, many of them the diseases of poverty, made worse by poor education. I know that in some of the more remote rural areas around here, only about half of all five-year old children have had the full course of immunisations. Without them, they are at risk of diseases that by now have largely disappeared from my suburban London practice: polio, diphtheria, tetanus, whooping cough, measles, as well as tuberculosis.

Sitting in on a consultation with one of my Cuban colleagues, I think of Lady Margaret and all that multitude of 'chemical marriages' back in London – people like John and Amanda – then of Warren and his 'bad back', and of the hundreds of hours I've spent over the years on sniffles and colds, minor blemishes and invisible rashes, all those lengthy talks only about trivia, about the surface of things.

But there's nothing more to be said. We have to get back to Umtata before nightfall. After dark, this area can be a dangerous place.

It might be any sprawling shantytown outside of Cape Town – Khayelitsha, say – but it's not. And yet here are exactly the same ramshackle little houses of cardboard and corrugated iron, and a few of brick, stretching haphazardly away across the landscape. There is the same stench of raw sewage, and the heavy smog of wood and coal smoke, the same wind whistling among the shacks, rattling their fragile walls, the same absence of telephones and taxis and clean running water, the same exhausted look on the faces of the people, slumped in their doorways, the same tattered clothing. And in the distance, too, you can see the same affluent high-rises of the nearby city, with its rapidly spreading shopping malls, health clubs and expensive boutiques.

Only the profusion of television aerials from the shanty roofs tells you that you are somewhere else – and the sounds of samba and salsa blaring from the TV sets within, run from pirated electricity cables. This is certainly not Johannesburg or the Transkei. I am being shown around one of the *favelas*, or shantytowns, on the outskirts of Porto Alegre, a city of about two and a half million in the south of Brazil, in the state of Rio Grande do Sul. It's in the early 1990s, and my guide, Dr Carlos Grossman – a compassionate, witty and charismatic physician – is the founder of one of the most innovative health care programmes in all of Latin America.

His *servicio de saúde comuntaria*, or community health programme, run by dedicated doctors and nurses, brings primary health care to six or seven of the poorest *favelas* in town, with a combined population of about 70,000. It's run out of the Nosso Senhora da Conceição district hospital, but there's also a network of small clinics or 'health posts' (*poste de saúde*), like the Transkei health centre, run for about eight hours a day in each shantytown. For these people, the very poorest of the urban poor, Dr Grossman's system often provides the only health care that they will ever get.

He takes me round two of the most impoverished *favelas*: Vila Divina Providencia and Vila Floresta, and then to meet the staff of one of the local clinics. The clinic is rather similar to the health centre in the Transkei. It has the same feel about it, the same dedication and scarce resources. In both places you can see the same exhausted but elated look on the faces of the clinic staff. The young doctors, from all over Brazil, describe themselves to me as 'social doctors' – dedicated to health care, but also to community development. Each week they spend half their work hours helping the local people, improving their housing and roads, their sanitation and street-lighting. They run literacy programmes, women's groups, sports teams, even a puppet theatre for the children. They give classes on health education and teach first aid. They train locally recruited community health workers or 'health agents' (*agente de saúde*), mostly women, and mostly volunteers, to improve the health of their families as well as their community. Most importantly, they understand keenly the social context of illness, especially poverty, in ways that most British or American doctors no longer do. This is something important in a country like Brazil, so big and so unequal that it's no wonder that some economist has nicknamed it 'Bel-India' – Belgium and India. It's an uncomfortable combination of First and Third Worlds, with very little in-between.

Dr Grossman's *servicio*, like the health centre in the Transkei, shows me an example of a novel type of medicine, one with a much more open and co-operative relationship between doctor, patient and community. It's a triangular partnership very different from what I've become used to in sedate London suburban practice, or from what I've seen in the United States, both with their specialised roles, formal hierarchies, rigid division between doctor and patient, and over-reliance on expensive technology. There's a lesson here for any British or American doctor, for to me this engagement with a community seems more like *real* medicine, much more than techno-medicine could ever be. There's a different, engaged, raw type of medicine being practised here, at the very frontline of human suffering. It's a type of medicine that has always attracted me.

And in an environment where so many children die young, from much the same diseases as in the Transkei, there's no place for 'paper patients' here.

Only real ones.

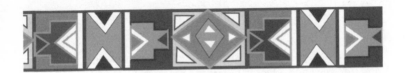

CHAPTER
24

The Brass Plaque

It is the very last day of the Medical Centre. Tomorrow it will be closed down after many years on this site, and the patients will reluctantly disperse to other practices nearby. Doctors and nurses and receptionists will all go their own separate ways. It's time to move on.

After 27 years in practice, both here and in other parts of London and in surrounding towns, it's time for me to leave clinical medicine for a while, to concentrate now on writing, and on teaching other doctors and medical students. One journey is ending; another is about to begin. But it's still tightly screwed to the outside wall of the building, that rectangular brass plaque mounted on a thick wooden base, the one with my name and all my university degrees engraved across it. To remove it, I have brought along most of my tool kit, as well as the whole bag of tools from my car, a full collection of pliers, chisels, screwdrivers, wrenches and drills, which together should do the trick. If I really cannot manage it myself, then I will just have to get a carpenter to rip it off for me. Either way, it has to come off today.

I put my screwdriver between it and the wall, and give a light, experimental, push. To my surprise, the plaque drops right off the wall and into my hand. Over the years the masonry below it seems to have become soft and powdery, and now crumbles easily and without any resistance.

It's almost as if it's been waiting for just this moment to be released.

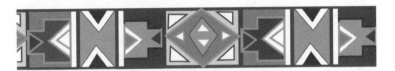

BIBLIOGRAPHY

I have listed here a number of books, journal articles and academic papers, organized by chapter, which I hope will be useful for further background on the particular subject of that chapter. I have also included some of my own academic papers and other publications.

Preface
Brody, Howard (2003) *Stories of Sickness* (2nd edition). New York: Oxford University Press.

Doyle, Arthur Conan (1963) *Tales of Adventure and Medical Life.* London: John Murray.

Helman, C.G. (2003) Physician Writers: Cecil Helman. *The Lancet* **361**, 2252.

Helman, C.G. (1981) General Practitioner as Social Anthropologist, *British Medical Journal* **282**, 787-788.

Kleinman, Arthur (1988) *The Illness Narratives.* New York: Basic Books.

Konner, Melvyn (1993) *Medicine at the Crossroads.* London: BBC Books.

Remen, Rachel Naomi (2000) *My Grandfather's Blessings.* New York: Riverhead Books.

Selzer, Richard (1996) *Letters to a Young Doctor.* New York: Harcourt Brace & Company.

Asylums
Laing, R.D. (1967) *The Politics of Experience and The Bird of Paradise.* Harmondsworth: Penguin.

Weiss, Peter (1965) *Marat .* London: Calder & Boyars.

Medical School
Bickford-Smith, V., van Heyningen, E. & Worden, M. (1999) *Cape*

Town in the Twentieth Century. Cape Town: David Philip Publishers

Helman, Cecil. (1992) *The Body Of Frankenstein's Monster: Essays in Myth and Medicine.* New York: W.W. Norton. See Chapter 8: 'The Dissecting Room', pp. 114-123.

Louw, Jan H. (1969) *In the Shadow Table Mountain: A History of the University of Cape Town Medical School.* Cape Town: Struik.

Sparks, Allister (1990) *The Mind of South Africa.* London: Heinemann.

UNESCO (1967) *Apartheid: Its effects on education, science, culture and information.* Paris: UNESCO.

Side-Show

Bogdan, Robert (1988) *Freak Show.* Chicago: University of Chicago Press.

Cassell, Eric J. (1976) *The Healer's Art..* New York: J.B. Lippincott.

Howell, Michael & Ford, Peter (1980) *The True History of the Elephant Man.* Harmondsworth: Penguin Books.

UNESCO (1967) *Apartheid: Its effects on education, science, culture and information.* Paris: UNESCO.

Casualties

Jeffrey, Roger (2001) Normal rubbish: deviant patients in casualty departments. In: Davey, B, Gray, A. & Seale, C. (Eds.)*Health and Disease; A Reader (3rd Edition).* Milton Keynes: Open University Press, pp. 363-368.

The Green Mask

Cassell, Joan (1986) 'Dismembering the Image of God': Surgeons, Heroes, Wimps and Miracles. *Anthropology Today*, **2**(2), 13-15.

Cassell, Joan (1991) *Expected Miracles: Surgeons at Work.* Philadelphia: Temple University Press.

Eliade, Mircea (1986) Masks: Mythical and Religious Origins. In: Apostolas-Cappdona, Diane (ed.) *Symbols, the Sacred, and the Arts.* New York: Crossroads, pp. 64-71.

Eliade, Mircea (1989) *Shamanism: Archaic Techniques of Ecstasy.* London: Arkana .

Katz, Pearl (1981) Ritual in the operating room. *Ethnology* **20**, 335-50.

Rosman, Abraham & Rubel, Paula G. (1990) Structural patterning in

Kwakiutl art and literature. *MAN: Journal of the Royal Anthropological Institute.* **25**, 620-640.

London

Helman, Cecil G. (2001) *Culture, Health and Illness* (4th edition). London: Hodder Arnold.

Keesing, R.M. & Strathern, A. (1997) *Cultural Anthropology: A Contemporary Perspective.* Fort Worth: Harcourt Brace College Publishers.

Kleinman, Arthur (1988) *Rethinking Psychiatry.* New York: Free Press.

Peacock, James L. (1986) *The Anthropological Lens.* Cambridge: Cambridge University Press.

Possession

Douglas, Mary (ed.) (1970) *Witchcraft Confessions and Accusations.* London: Tavistock.

Helman, Cecil G. (1986) 'Feed a Cold, Starve a Fever': Folk models of infection in an English suburban community, and their relation to medical treatment. In: Currer, Caroline & Stacey, Meg (eds.) *Concepts of Health, Illness and Disease.* Lymington Spa: Berg Publishers, pp. 213-234.

Helman, Cecil (2003) Natural History: Changing Folk Perceptions of Health and Disease. In: Boon, T. & Jones, I. (eds.) *Treat Yourself: Health Consumers in a Medical Age.* London: Science Museum, pp. 9-11.

Helman, Cecil G. (2004) Possession: On Being a Doctor. *Annals of Internal Medicine* **140** (3), 229-230.

Lewis, Ioan M. (1971) *Ecstatic Religion.* Harmondsworth: Penguin.

Porter, Roy (1966) What is Disease? In: Porter, Roy (ed.) (1996) *The Cambridge Illustrated History of Medicine.* Cambridge: Cambridge University Press, pp. 82-117.

Porter, Roy (Ed.) (1985) *Patients and Practitioners: Lay perceptions of medicine in pre-industrial society.* Cambridge: Cambridge University Press.

Sontag, Susan (1979) *Illness as Metaphor.* New York: Vintage.

Trevor-Roper, Hugh R. (1969) *The European Witch-Craze of the 16th and 17th Centuries.* Harmondsworth: Penguin.

Déformation Professionelle

Helman, C.G. (2000) Dr Chameleon. *British Journal of General Practice* **50**, 524.

The Illusion of Doubles

Capgras, J. & Reboul-Lachaux (1923) Illusion des 'sosies' dans un délire systématise chronique. *Bulletine de la Société Clinique de Médecine Mental* **2**, 6-16.

Dostoyevsky, Fyodor (1972) *Notes from the Underground/The Double.* Translated by Jessie Coulson. Harmondsworth: Penguin Books.

Eco, Umberto (1986) *Travels in Hyperreality.* New York: Harcourt Brace Jovanovich.

Todd, J, Dewhurst, K. & Wallis, G. (1981) The syndrome of Capgras. *British Journal of Psychiatry* **139**, 319-327.

Boundaries

Cassell, Eric J. (1976) *The Healer's Art.* New York: J.B. Lippincott.

McDougall, Joyce (1989) *Theatres of the Body.* London: Free Association Books.

Remen, Rachel Naomi (1996) *Kitchen Table Wisdom.* New York: Riverhead Books.

Remen, Rachel Naomi (2000) *My Grandfather's Blessings.* New York: Riverhead Books.

Prescriptions

Benson, Herbert (1996) *Timeless Healing: The Power and Biology of Belief.* New York: Simon and Schuster.

Helman, C.G. (1986) 'Tonic', 'Fuel' and 'Food': Social and symbolic aspects of the long-term use of psychotropic drugs. In: Gabe, Jonathan & Williams, Paul (eds.) *Tranquillisers: Social, Psychological, and Clinical Perspectives.* London: Tavistock, pp. 199-226.

Membranes

Gordon, Deborah R. (1990) Embodying illness, embodying cancer. *Culture, Medicine and Psychiatry* **14**, 275-97.

Sontag, Susan (1979) *Illness as Metaphor.* New York: Vintage.

Sontag, Susan (1988) *AIDS and Its Metaphors.* New York: Farrar Strauss Giroux.

An Autumn Leaf

Helman, C.G. (1997) The Role of Culture in Medical Education. *Changing Medical Education and Medical Practice* (World Health Organization), No. 11, pp. 24-25, July 1997.

Obeyesekere, G. (1977) The theory and practice of Ayurvedic medicine. *Culture, Medicine and Psychiatry* 1, 155-81.

Qureshi, Bashir. (1990) Alternative/Complementary Medicine. In: McAvoy, B.R. & Donaldson, L.J. (eds.) *Health Care for Asians.* Oxford: Oxford University Press, pp. 93-116.

Srinavasan, P. (1995) National health policy for traditional medicine in India. *World Health Forum* 16, 190-195.

Grand Rounds

Hastings, Paul (1976) *Medicine: An International History.* London: Ernest Benn.

Pickstone, Jon (1996) Medicine, Society, and the State. In: Porter, Roy (ed.) *The Cambridge Illustrated History of Medicine.* Cambridge: Cambridge University Press, pp. 304-341.

Shorter, Edward (1996) Primary Care. In: Porter, Roy (ed.) *The Cambridge Illustrated History of Medicine.* Cambridge: Cambridge University Press, pp. 118-153.

Stevens, Rosemary (2001) The evolution of the health-care systems in the United States and the United Kingdom: similarities and differences. In: Davey, B, Gray, A. & Seale, C (eds.) *Health and Disease; A Reader* (3rd Edition). Milton Keynes: Open University Press, pp. 319-325.

Healing Time

Bannister, Anthony (1988) *The Bushmen.* Cape Town: Struik.

Byng-Hall, John (1988) Scripts and legends in families and family therapy. *Family Process* 27, 167-79.

Helman, Cecil (ed.) (2003) *Doctors and Patients: An Anthology.* Oxford: Radcliffe Medical Press. See: Helman, Cecil:' Introduction: The Healing Bond', pp. 1-14.

Helman, Cecil G. (2005) Cultural aspects of time and ageing, *EMBO Reports* (European Molecular Biology Organization) Vol 6 (Special Issue), S54-S58.

Lewis-Williams, D. & Pearce, D. (2004) *San Spirituality.* Cape Town:

Double Storey.

Like, Robert C., Rogers J. & McGoldrick, Monica (1988) Reading and interpreting genograms: a systematic approach. *Journal of Family Practice* **26** (4), 407-412.

Prince-Embury, S (1984) The family health tree: a form of identifying physical symptom patterns within the family. *Journal of Family Practice* **18**, 75-81.

Shorter, Edward (1996) Primary Care. In: Porter, Roy (ed.) *The Cambridge Illustrated History of Medicine*. Cambridge: Cambridge University Press, pp. 118-153.

Hospital

Ofri, Danielle (2005) *Incidental Findings: Lessons from My Patients in the Art of Medicine*. Boston: Beacon Press,

Porter, Roy (1996) Hospitals and Surgery. In: Porter, Roy (ed.) *The Cambridge Illustrated History of Medicine*. Cambridge: Cambridge University Press, pp. 202-245.

Sacks, Oliver (1984) *A Leg To Stand On*. London & New York: Picador.

Woodhandler, S., Himmelstein, D.U. & Lewontin, J.P. (1993) Administrative costs in US hospitals. *New England Journal of Medicine* **329**, 400-403.

Paradigm Lost

Doyle, Arthur Conan (1963) *Tales of Adventure and Medical Life*. London: John Murray.

Helman, C.G. (1991) Limits of Biomedical Explanation, *The Lancet* **337**, 1079-1083

Helman, Cecil (2002) Editorial: The culture of general practice. *British Journal of General Practice* **52** (481), 619-620.

Louw, Jan H. (1969) *In the Shadow Table Mountain: A History of the University of Cape Town Medical School*. Cape Town: Struik.

Kleinman, Arthur (1988) *The Illness Narratives*. New York: Basic Books.

Konner, Melvyn (1993) *The Trouble With Medicine*. London: BBC Books.

Porter, Roy (ed.) (1966) Chapter 6, Hospitals and Surgery. In: *The Cambridge Illustrated History of Medicine*. Cambridge: Cambridge University Press.

Shamans

Brown, Diana D. (1994) *Umbanda.* New York: Columbia University Press.

Halifax, Joan (1979) *Shamanic Voices.* Harmondsworth, Penguin.

Helman, Cecil G. (2001) *Culture, Health and Illness* (4th Edition). London: Hodder Arnold, pp. 50-78.

Kossoy, Edward & Ohry, Abraham (1992) *The Feldshers.* Jerusalem: Magnes Press.

Lewis, Ioan M. (1971) *Ecstatic Religion.* Harmondsworth: Penguin.

Turner, Victor W. (1964) An Ndembu doctor in practice. In: Kiev, Ari (ed.) *Magic, Faith and Healing.* New York: Free Press, pp. 230-263.

Turner, Victor W. (1969) *The Ritual Process.* Harmondsworth: Penguin.

Vitebsky, Piers (1995) *The Shaman.* London: Macmillan.

World Health Organisation (1978) *The Promotion and Development of Traditional Medicine* (WHO Technical Report Series 622). Geneva: World Health Organisation

World Health Organisation (2002) *WHO Traditional Medicine Strategy 2002-2005.* Geneva: World Health Organisation.

Placebos

Benson, H. & Epstein, M.D. (1975) The placebo effect: a neglected asset in the care of patients. *Journal of the American Medical Association* **232**, 1225-1227.

Benson, Herbert (1996) *Timeless Healing: The Power and Biology of Belief.* New York: Simon and Schuster.

Hahn, R.A. (1997) The nocebo phenomenon: concept, evidence, and implications for public health. *Preventive Medicine* **26**, 607-611.

Helman, Cecil G. (2001) Placebos and nocebos: the cultural construction of belief. In: Peters, David (ed.) *Understanding the Placebo Effect in Complementary Medicine.* Edinburgh: Churchill Livingstone. pp. 3-16.

Kienle, G.S. & Kiene, H. (2001) A critical reanalysis of the concept, magnitude and existence of placebo effects. In: Peters, D. (ed.) *Understanding the Placebo Effect in Complementary Medicine: Theory, Practice and Research.* London: Churchill Livingstone, pp. 31-50.

Lex, Barbara (1977) Voodoo death: New thoughts on an old explanation. In: Landy, D. (ed.) *Culture, Disease and Healing: Studies in Medical Anthropology.* New York: Macmillan, pp. 327-331.

Turner, Victor (1969) *The Ritual Process.* Harmondsworth: Penguin.

Third Worlds

Gray, Alastair (ed.) (1993) *World Health and Disease.* Milton Keynes: Open University Press.

Haines, Andrew & Helman, Cecil (1990) Anglo-Brazilian link in general practice. *RCGP Connection,* Issue 4, pp. 3-4.

Harpham, T, Lusty, T. & Vaughan, P. (eds.) (1988) *In the Shadow of the City: Community Health and the Urban Poor.* Oxford: Oxford University Press.

Helman, Cecil G. (2001) *Culture, Health and Illness* (4th Edition) London: Hodder Arnold, pp. 50-78.

Helman, Cecil & Yogeswaran, Parimalani (2004) Perceptions of childhood immunizations in rural Transkei: a qualitative study. *South African Medical Journal* **94** (2), 835-838.

Mahlalela, X., Rohde, J., Meidany, F., Hutchinson, P. & Bennett, J. (2000) *Primary Health Care in the Eastern Cape Province.* Pretoria, South Africa: The Equity Project.

World Health Organisation (1995) *The World Health Report 1995 – Bridging the Gaps.* Geneva: World Health Organisation.

Also from Hammersmith Press

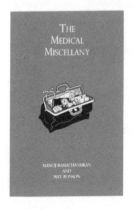

The Medical Miscellany
By Manoj Ramachandran & Max Ronson
174 pp £9.99
ISBN: 1-905140-05-3
Published 17 August 2005

This fascinating collection of medically-related items will inform, tantalize and infuriate you by turns. How can you tell if a murder victim was left- or right-handed? How many euphemisms can you think of for unmentionable parts of the body? What has chicken pox got to do with chickens? And does a famous doctor or medical scientist share your birthday?

We challenge you not to find something unexpected on every page, nor to smile or groan at almost every entry. How much do you know? How much will you be able to remember?

About Hammersmith Press Ltd

An independent publisher providing books on matters relating to diet, health and illness for the non-specialist reader.

Hammersmith Press is a new publishing house producing books for the general public and health professionals that promote better health and well being through a greater understanding of the functioning of the human body and mind.

Founded in 2004 we see a need for books that address readers as interested, intelligent custodians of their own health and who want to have thorough explanations of the advice they are given rather than taking guidance on trust.

For many of our readers, modern Western medicine offers important solutions but is often not sufficient in the face of the uncertainties and suffering associated with illness and death. We are proud to publish *Suburban Shaman*, which asks us, doctors and patients alike, never 'to medicalise the human condition' or 'casually to convert everyday problems into medical diagnoses', but to understand the broader role we ask doctors to take on as healers, whether or not they can cure us.